SCIENCE OF ENERGY FLOW®

FOOT REFLEXOLOGY WITH HERBAL STRESS RELIEF

Also by Dr. Martha Libster

The Nurse Herbalist:
Integrative Insights for Holistic Practice

Enlightened Charity:
The Holistic Nursing Care, Education,
and Advices Concerning the Sick
of Sister Matilda Coskery, 1799-1870

Herbal Diplomats:
The Contribution of Early American Nurses
(1830–1860) to Nineteenth-Century Health Care
Reform and the Botanical Medical Movement

The Bamboo Bridge:
www.BambooBridge.org

Demonstrating Care: The Art of Integrative Nursing

The Integrative Herb Guide for Nurses
(Book and CD-ROM with videos)

SCIENCE OF ENERGY FLOW®

Foot Reflexology with Herbal Stress Relief

DR. MARTHA M. LIBSTER

GOLDEN APPLE PUBLICATIONS

Cover/Illustrations/Book Design: Mark Gelotte www.markgelotte.com
Copy Edit: Rose Foley
Photography: Juliana Cesano

Printed in the United States

Library of Congress Control Number: 2014941756

Includes bibliographical references and Index

ISBN 9780975501856

Libster, Martha Mathews 1960-

1. Reflexology 2. Massage 3. Self Care 4. Herbal Medicine
5. Stress Management 6. Foot Zone Therapy I. Title: Science of Energy Flow

Thank you, Divine Mother

ACKNOWLEDGMENTS AND GRATITUDE

Thank you to all of my family, friends, patients, clients, and students who have come to under-stand the simple elegance of foot reflexology with herbal applications as one of the finest expressions of the science and art of healing. Your enthusiasm and your feet inspire me! I am grateful for the opportunity and the privilege to share this wisdom tradition in its entirety in the clinic, classroom, and now in this little book. While I fully acknowledge that our comprehension of holographic science is still in its infancy, I am hopeful that *Science of Energy Flow® Foot Reflexology with Herbal Stress Relief* will allow us to engage in greater dialog about it. With each treatment over these past thirty years, I have become more and more aware of holographic science as a key to grasping the full beauty of the power within us to heal ourselves and care for others. It took me three decades to get to a point where I felt I could begin to express that beauty in the words of a book. The support I have received for this book affirms the work and encourages and humbles me to continue on despite our scientific ambiguities. For those who are now coming to the work, let me share what my teachers told me early on: "If you're not sure about the 'water,' just put your toes in first." Put everything to the test of your own awareness and give it a try!

To all who have made this book possible – my teachers now passed away but long remembered – I thank you. For those who have made this book beautiful – Harold, Mark, Rose, Juliana, Julie, and Sandy – I thank you from the center of my heart.

My love for the science and art of energy flow and the feet is a result of the dance. I have been a dancer since I was seven years old when I was first trained in the American Denishawn dance tradition, thanks to Margot Gillis. As all good teachers of this ancient non-verbal art form are wont to do, Margot provided the literal stage for my spiritual development in early life. I first learned about energy flow by observing, experiencing, and incorporating movement in my own body and interpreting musical rhythms, cadence, and phrasing according to the flow of emotion through my muscles and bones. I also remember my first observations of energy fields around people when moving on stage while being lit in violet light from below—a typical lighting design used in the dance. I used my fingers to trace light patterns in the air and never wondered how I knew where the other dancers were on stage. The dance experience enabled me to use my kinesthetic senses and develop keen perceptions of space and its occupants.

It was also in the dance that I gained a love for feet. I learned that proper shoes were important to health as well as the ability to dance, and did not complain when I had only one or two tie shoes to choose from for my school shoes when other kids were wearing the newest fashion with buckles or straps. I first learned to take special care of my feet when I advanced to dancing *en pointe* in shoes that made my toes hurt even though they were lined with rabbit fur or lamb's wool. Later, I would often dance barefoot with a modern dance company in New York City. While my partner for one of the dances and I were sitting on the floor during a rehearsal, I mentioned that I had a headache. Strangely, she grabbed one of my feet and started pressing her thumb and knuckles into my foot. Although dancers are trained to endure physical pain, particularly in their feet, what she did hurt!

I remember quietly squirming away from her grasp and asking her what the heck she was doing. Her answer: "reflexology." Hours later, I could only remember that experience of pain as helpful to my energy level and my performance.

She had convinced me that reflexology might help my headache, so I let her twist my toes and press more. Not only did my tension headache clear, but when I got up to dance, I was really "on my legs." I felt so centered that I was able to do four or five turns at a point in the music where I had previously done one or two. I was hooked after that powerful experience. Not long afterward, I found myself talking with colleagues in the healing arts world about performing the ritual of the washing of the feet—something I had learned from my father, a Christian minister. It took a few years, but I got my wish to work with feet when I met and subsequently apprenticed with Oma in 1984. Foot reflexology was Oma's specialty. It was her life work. My calling to foot reflexology and washing the feet started with a dream I had involving amethyst stones and visions of a practice in healing touch. When Oma came to the door of her clinic in Glendale, California, she was wearing a large amethyst pendant and her hands were strong from decades of healing practice.

Oma and I spent two years together in the clinic on the days when I was not studying to be a nurse. My nursing career has always been touched and influenced by traditional healers and healing traditions as well as nurses. This book includes the foundational teachings I received from Oma and, subsequently, other master healer-teachers. I hope to honor the memory of my teachers, who are all gone now to the spirit world.

While I appreciate and have participated willingly in the call to scientific research and writing as a nurse and health care historian, this book is a joyful departure for me. It is a recording of the teachings of reflexology and related healing traditions as I learned them from my teachers and as they have evolved in my care as a dancer, nurse, herbalist, and historian. I have trademarked this tradition as the Science of Energy Flow® Foot Reflexology (SEF) out of my love for historic preservation and a desire to protect and root the oral traditions passed to me in written form as carefully and completely as possible.

It is never a simple task to translate oral tradition into the written word. What I have provided here is my best attempt to capture the essence or spirit as well as action of the teaching as it is embodied in this work as a healing service to people. I am the first to admit my belief that "actions speak louder than words" and that a "picture is worth a thousand words." This belief is why I have taught SEF rather than written about it all these years. But as in all of my service to students, the question compels the answer. It is clear that the time has come to provide a written guide for those who will *flow* with this teaching. The artwork, the charts, and the content provided here are what I believe to be "progressive revelation" respectful of tradition as taught by my teachers. It is my hope that you, the reader, will find this step-by-step guidebook progressive and revealing. It is also my vision that in this book you will find a tradition familiar to you in its fundamental simplicity and yet challenging in its scientific call to expand your awareness and perceptions of new dimensions of health, healing, and the joy of being alive with greater *under-standing*.

Martha Mathews Libster
Illinois, USA 2014

EDITOR'S NOTE

This book *Science of Energy Flow*® is meant to sound like Dr. Martha is having a conversation with the reader. To that end, we've taken liberties with certain grammatical constructions to give the book a more informal feel. Specifically, we frequently use "they" as a singular pronoun and "their" as a singular modifier rather than the more customary, but often awkward, "he/she," "his/her," or plural possessive constructions. Our overall intent is to be mindful about our approach so as to make the book as accessible and readily understood as possible—and that intention extends to grammar as well.

CONTENTS

◈

A Re-introduction to Your Under-Standing

Take a break and put your feet up! Now take a really good look at your feet. Where have your feet been? What do your feet "say" about you? Why care for your feet anyway? They're just feet…right? What do you see when you look at your feet? Whatever it is, I guarantee that after reading this book, you will never perceive your feet in the same way again! So, take a good look now and get ready for an experience in the healing arts and sciences like *no other.*

The Science of Energy Flow® Foot Reflexology (SEF) is a unique gentle remedy. This book reveals SEF as a healing science grounded in time-honored practice patterns, contemporary research, and a palette of numerous touch and visualization techniques that you apply when helping yourself and others realize greater health and well being. Stories from my experiences in practice provide the context for the illustration of a healing art form that can seem elusive. But once you experience SEF and begin to study the practice, you may come to find it quite familiar. SEF incorporates ancient healing traditions as well as new scientific understanding. To work with the feet is to work with a person's *under-standing*—literally. You will come to know this work with the understanding as more than a simple foot massage. SEF can activate your divine blueprint for wholeness, body memory, and the unconscious dreams many people hold for a flowing future of peace as well as healing of body, mind, and spirit. If these words seem a bit lofty, I apologize. Just know that I have seen it happen time and again. SEF can inspire healing and peace. This book explains how. It is a step-by-step guide that you can apply when caring for yourself and for others.

The scientific premise of this book is that health, healing, and peace are the natural result of energy flow directed in service to humanity. It is the culmination of my 30 years of caring for people in a way that frees the energy flow of body, mind, emotion, and spirit by simply working the feet! This book contains a collection of stories of healing and peace that extend from one simple intention to promote the free flow of energy. Both the healer and the recipient of healing engage in the exchange of energy that facilitates healing or change that is precipitated by the free flow of energy. Free or harmonious flow of energy is the definition of health in many cultures. The notion that "disease" is actually the manifestation of a blockage or stagnation of energy dates back centuries, such as in Asian healing tradition. It is still a powerful focal point of Eastern healing today.

One important first step to gaining a good understanding of what constitutes a free flow of energy through the body and its organs and systems is to study anatomy and physiology. Human anatomy is the study of the form and structures of the body, such as bones and organs. Physiology is the study of the function of the body. It is in the study of physiology that we begin to comprehend the flow of energy through the body and what distinguishes free flow or healthy flow through a specific anatomical structure and what constitutes stagnant flow that can result in disease. Asian peoples have spent centuries exploring and defining the flow of energy in the body as a whole and its organs and systems. Energy flow is known in Asian tradition as *chi* or *qi*. The word not only refers to the substance of energy but also denotes flow of energy. Therefore, the term qi will be used interchangeably with energy flow throughout this book.

Qi is a term that is quite well known around the globe. Eastern philosophies of the healing arts have migrated to the West for some time. East-West cultural exchange in the healing arts has been important to the promotion of global peace. Many spiritual teachers have been leaders in the East-West exchange. One of them, Swami Sri Yukteswar, sent Paramahansa Yogananda to the United States to cultivate knowledge of the science and spirit of yoga, specifically Kriya Yoga. This 1920 diplomatic mission left an indelible mark on history. Today, yoga is a household term in the West while in the early twentieth century it was not. Despite the steady development of understanding of yoga and qi in the West, some people continue to distrust Eastern philosophy and science.

SEF, with its cultural roots in ancient Eastern and Egyptian traditions, has also been misunderstood, misrepresented and, at times, maligned. On November 4, 1991, the following was published in *Time* magazine:

> Many alternative therapies assume that mind and body are subtly interlocked and influence each other powerfully. In terms of credibility, they run the gamut from the generally accepted—acupuncture for pain relief; to the plausible—inhaling eucalyptus to open the sinuses (aromatherapy); to the frankly bizarre—having the middle of your foot manipulated to improve liver function (reflexology).

At the time, the term "alternative medicine" had been created by biomedicine to describe healing modalities that were not taught in medical schools. Biomedical publications painted a picture of many of these modalities as new to the healing arts, specifically the practice of medicine. Anything new, any change, is perceived as a threat by the brain. New things can seem bizarre. But many if not most modalities, now referred to as "complementary therapies" in the biomedical culture, are actually not new. These modalities, which I prefer to refer to as "healing traditions," often are quite ancient or have their roots in ancient healing practices and systems.

In terms of SEF, while holographic science and explanations for how reflexology works may be "new," foot reflexology practice is not. Etched into the wall of the ancient Egyptian tomb of Ankhm'ahor dating back to the Sixth Dynasty is a relief [*See Figure 0-1*] showing people in profile giving and receiving touch treatment to the feet and hands. In the Bible, John 13 : 5-17, Jesus demonstrates the ritual of the washing of the feet while teaching his disciples principles from the ancient healing tradition. This traditional knowledge and the healing rituals will be discussed in greater detail throughout the book. The washing of the feet includes a healing ritual known as ablution. It is one of the most important techniques you will learn in SEF later in Chapter 1.

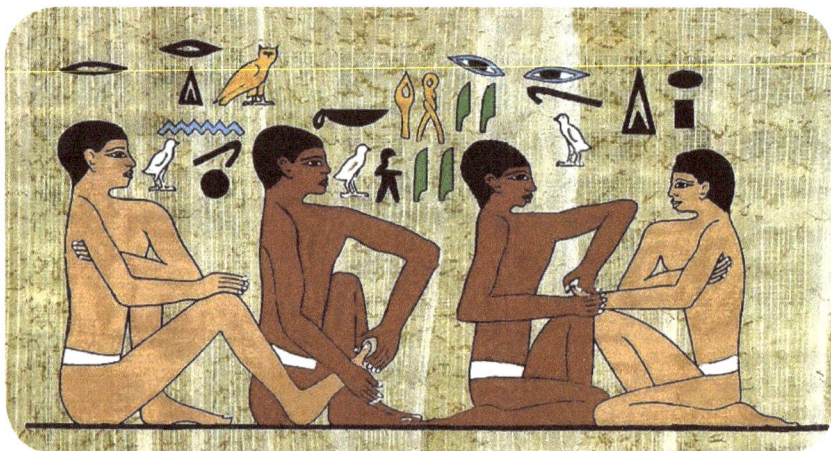

0-1 EGYPTIAN RELIEF

MEET THE FEET!

An understanding of suffering as part of human experience is universal as is awareness of a quest for health and healing. SEF holds the potential to relieve suffering and promote health and healing through the feet, which are our *under-standing*. Let's begin with your own feet first. Sit in a chair with your back supported so that you can sit upright comfortably. Look at your bare feet on the floor. Then place your right foot over your left knee or on a chair in front of

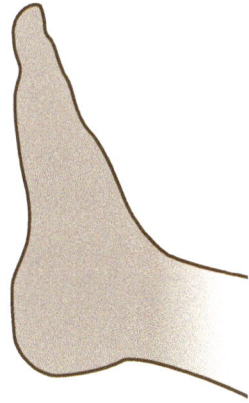

0-2   SEATED FORM

you so that you can view the whole foot from the side. [*See Figure 0-2*] If you look at the inner side of your foot in a vertical position with toes pointed upward as in the illustration, you will notice that the foot, in this position, looks like a seated person. The toes are the head. This can be a bit sketchy at first, but as you gaze at your foot your perception may change. You may start to notice more features of the seated form in the foot.

Perception is a powerful tool. Here is an experiment that will show you what I mean. Count the F's you see in Figure 0-3:

FINISHED FILES ARE THE RESULT OF YEARS OF SCIENTIFIC STUDY COMBINED WITH THE EXPERIENCE OF MANY YEARS.

0-3   COUNT THE F's

5

I have shown this experiment as a slide at conferences and asked people to simply count the F's that they see. On the count of three, I ask them to call out the number of F's that they see. People call out numbers from two to six. There are actually six F's in the sentence and yet few people see all six F's. This experiment really causes people to think about perception and the mind. This experiment shows that we may not always see what is right in front of us or, in the case of our feet, what is underneath us that carries us day by day.

The two feet, together and side by side, are a full representation or what one of my teachers, Dr. Charles Ersdal of Norway, referred to specifically as the "entirety" of the human body with all of its systems, organs, and energy pathways. [*See Figure 0-4*] It is important that the eye and all of the senses as well as the mind be trained to perceive the two feet as an entirety. The reason for this is because the body and all of its systems, organs, and energy pathways are a whole. We care for others and ourselves as whole beings because all of the parts of ourselves are interrelated. The energy patterns of those inter-relationships become clearer as one works within this scientific system of understanding known as holographic science.

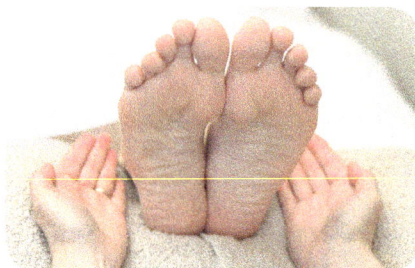

0-4 ENTIRETY

6

THE HOLOGRAM OF HUMAN ANATOMY

In SEF, the body, with all of its structures and organs (anatomy) and systems or processes (physiology), is represented or projected in its entirety in the feet. Both feet side by side are a hologram of human anatomy, a scaled-down version of the human body with all of its structures and systems. A hologram, simply stated, is a three-dimensional image formed by interference from a light source. Each part of the hologram holds within it a blueprint for replicating the whole. The first key to effecting a healing action through SEF lies in the ability to identify how each part of the hologram of the body is represented in feet that can be of any size—from baby feet to large adult feet. Reflexologists have worked over the decades to better define the positioning and placement of anatomical structures and systems within the hologram of the feet. This work is depicted in reflexology charts. The chart used in SEF is included here. [*See Figure 0-5*] This chart is the result of my work in anatomy and physiology, foot reflexology, and Foot Zone Therapy as well as what I have learned from treating hundreds of pairs of feet of all shapes and sizes since 1984. The effect of the accuracy of foot reflexology charts can be compared with the accuracy of a map. A person following a map that contains errors may very well make it to their destination. While they may not be harmed per se, they may spend more energy on getting back on the path than if they had a proper map in the first place. This is the issue with reflexology charts. Inaccuracies and underdeveloped charts do not necessarily harm someone, but they can delay proper treatment and healing.

Reflexology charts also represent the development of scientific knowledge of the hologram and, therefore, should demonstrate progress in our understanding of the placement of body organs and systems. The most accurate charts I have found to date are the charts

7

SCIENCE OF ENERGY FLOW®
SEF FOOT REFLEXOLOGY CHART

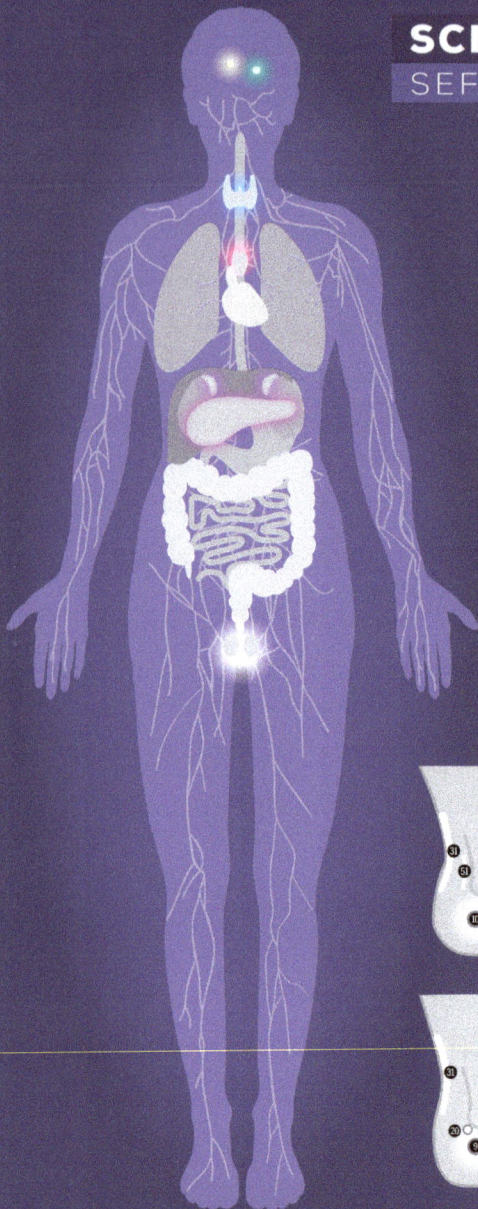

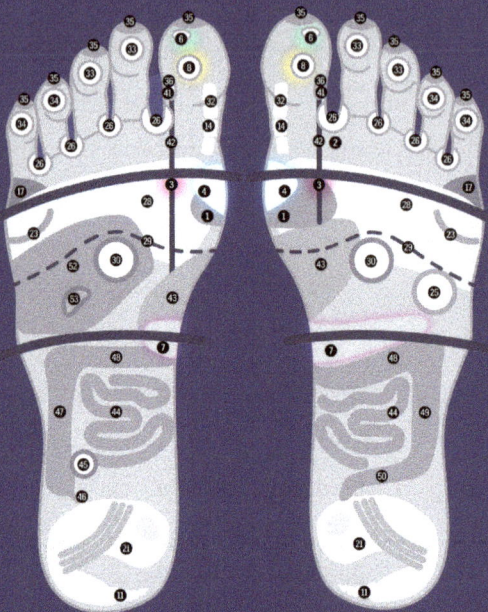

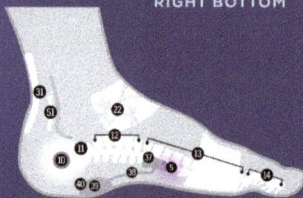

RIGHT BOTTOM

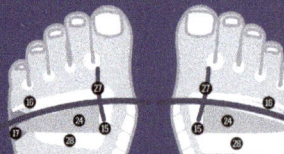

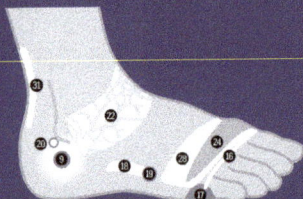

LEFT BOTTOM

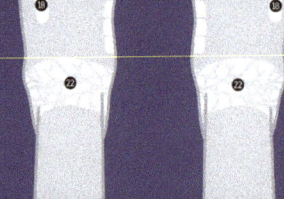

1.	HEART	14.	SPINE – CERVICAL
2.	AORTIC ARCH	15.	STERNUM
3.	HEART CHAKRA – THYMUS GLAND	16.	CLAVICLES
4.	THROAT CHAKRA – THYROID GLAND	17.	SHOULDERS
5.	SOLAR PLEXUS CHAKRA – ADRENAL GLANDS	18.	THIGHS
6.	THIRD EYE CHAKRA – PINEAL GLAND	19.	KNEES
7.	SEAT-OF-THE-SOUL CHAKRA – PANCREAS	20.	HIP JOINTS
8.	CROWN CHAKRA - PITUITARY GLAND	21.	PELVIS
9.	BASE CHAKRA – OVARIES/TESTES	22.	LYMPH CHANNELS – GROIN
10.	BASE CHAKRA – UTERUS/PROSTATE	23.	LYMPH – AXILLARY CHANNELS
11.	SPINE – COCCYX / SACRUM	24.	BREASTS
12.	SPINE –LUMBAR	25.	SPLEEN
13.	SPINE – THORACIC	26.	SINUSES / CERVICAL LYMPH DRAINAGE

27.	LARYNX / TRACHEA / BRONCHIOLES	41.	MOUTH/TONSILS
28.	LUNGS	42.	ESOPHAGUS
29.	DIAPHRAGM MUSCLE	43.	STOMACH
30.	SOLAR PLEXUS (NERVE CENTER)	44.	SMALL INTESTINE
31.	SCIATIC NERVE	45.	ILEOCECAL VALVE
32.	OCCIPUT / NECK	46.	APPENDIX
33.	EYES	47.	LARGE INTESTINE – ASCENDING COLON
34.	EARS	48.	LARGE INTESTINE – TRANSVERSE COLON
35.	HEAD / SKULL	49.	LARGE INTESTINE – DESCENDING COLON
36.	INNER EARS	50.	SIGMOID COLON
37.	KIDNEYS	51.	RECTUM
38.	URETERS	52.	LIVER
39.	BLADDER	53.	GALLBLADDER
40.	URETHRA		

Note: The SEF CHART is intended for support of the healing practice of pattern recognition of the energy fields of the body in its entirety, not the diagnosis of dise...

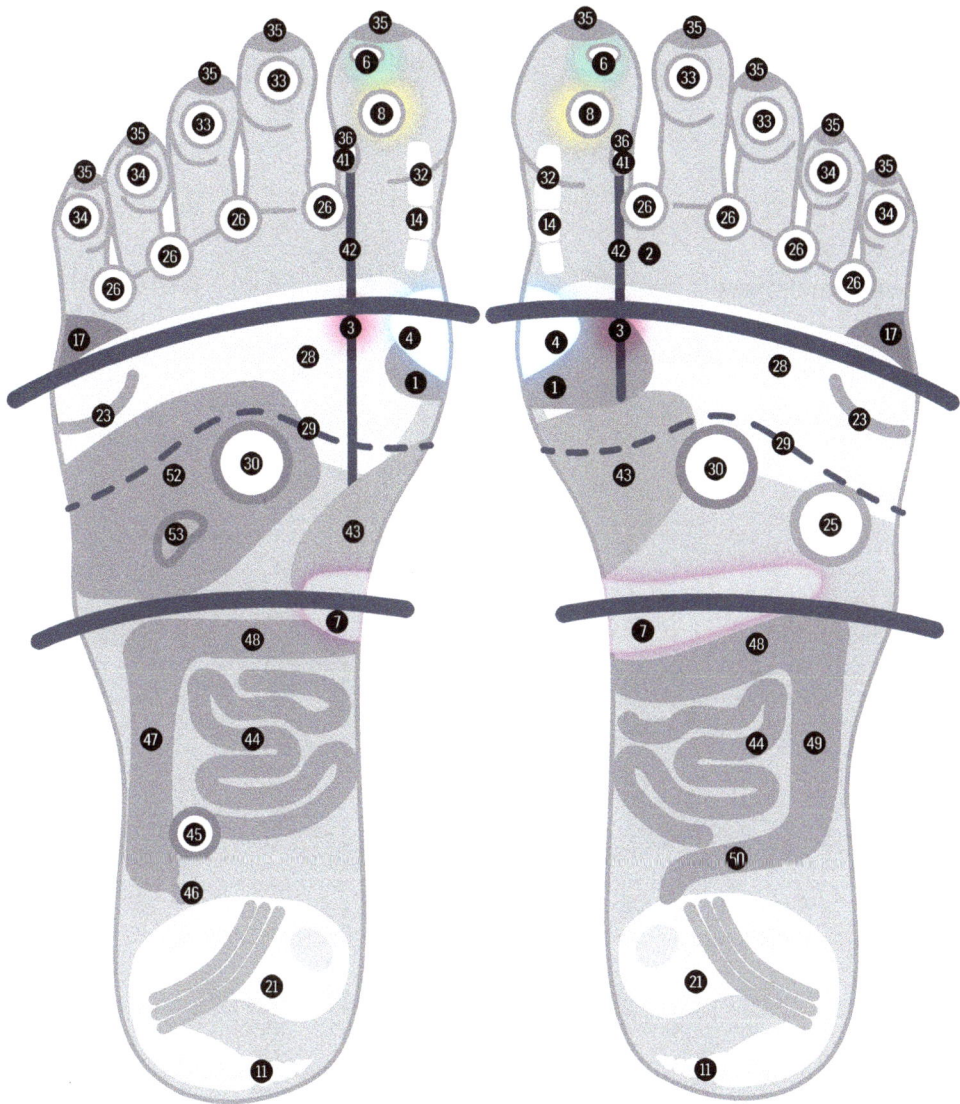

1. HEART
2. AORTIC ARCH
3. HEART CHAKRA - THYMUS GLAND
4. THROAT CHAKRA - THYROID GLAND
5. SOLAR PLEXUS CHAKRA - ADRENAL GLANDS
6. THIRD EYE CHAKRA - PINEAL GLAND
7. SEAT-OF-THE-SOUL CHAKRA - PANCREAS
8. CROWN CHAKRA - PITUITARY GLAND
9. BASE-OF-THE-SPINE CHAKRA - OVARIES/TESTES
10. BASE-OF-THE-SPINE CHAKRA - UTERUS/PROSTATE
11. SPINE- COCCYX / SACRUM
12. SPINE –LUMBAR
13. SPINE – THORACIC
14. SPINE – CERVICAL
15. STERNUM
16. CLAVICLE
17. SHOULDERS
18. THIGHS
19. KNEES
20. HIP JOINTS
21. PELVIS
22. LYMPH CHANNELS – GROIN
23. LYMPH CHANNELS – AXILLARY
24. BREASTS
25. SPLEEN
26. SINUS / CERVICAL LYMPH DRAINAGE
27. LARYNX / TRACHEA / BRONCHIOLES
28. LUNGS
29. DIAPHRAGM MUSCLE
30. SOLAR PLEXUS (NERVE CENTER)
31. SCIATIC NERVE
32. OCCIPUT / NECK
33. EYES
34. EARS
35. HEAD / SKULL
36. INNER EARS
37. KIDNEYS
38. URETERS
39. BLADDER
40. URETHRA
41. MOUTH/TONSILS
42. ESOPHAGUS
43. STOMACH
44. SMALL INTESTINE
45. ILEOCECAL VALVE
46. APPENDIX
47. LARGE INTESTINE – ASCENDING COLON
48. LARGE INTESTINE – TRANSVERSE COLON
49. LARGE INTESTINE – DESCENDING COLON
50. SIGMOID COLON
51. RECTUM
52. LIVER
53. GALLBLADDER

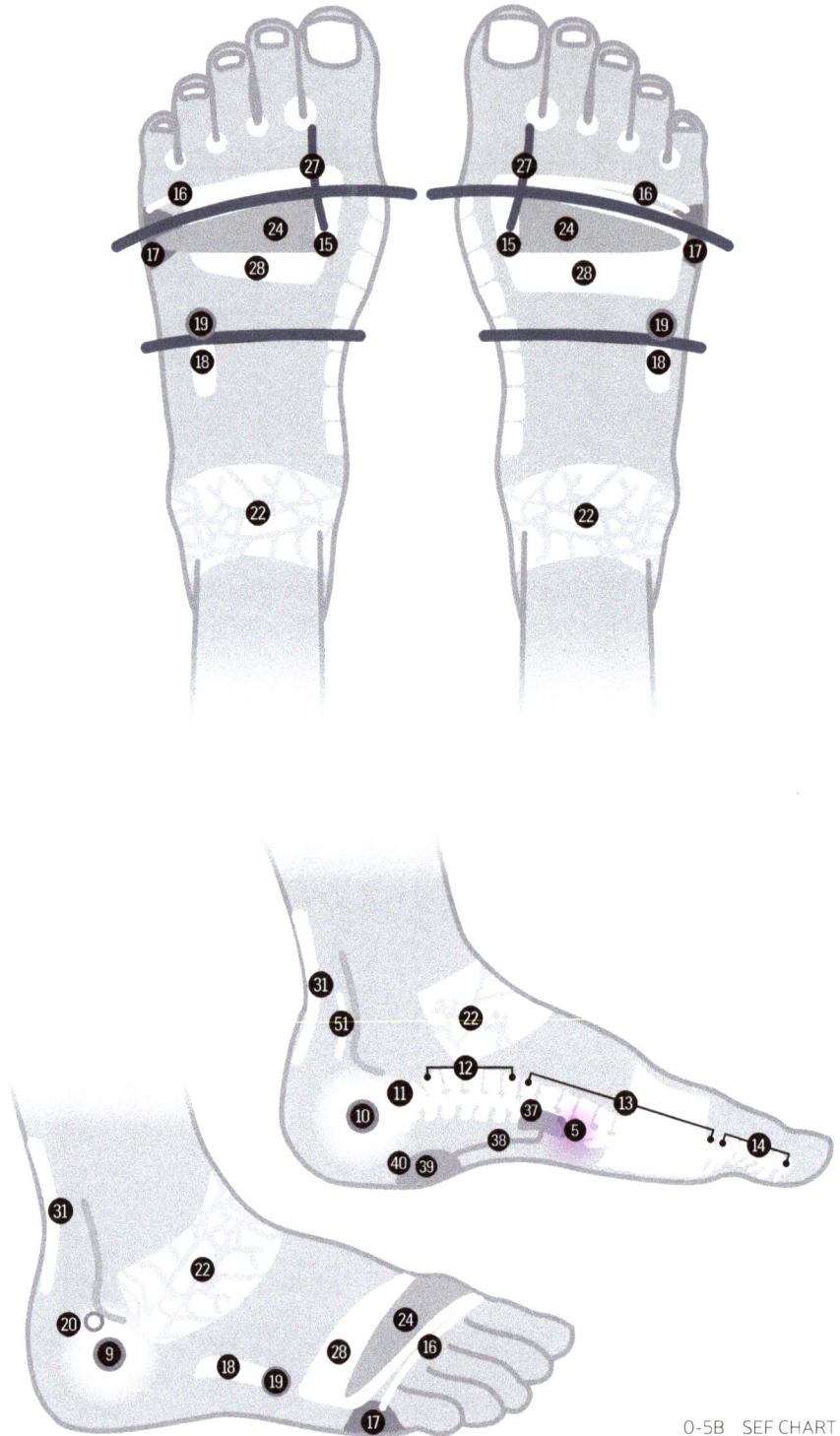

0-5B   SEF CHART

of Dr. Charles Ersdal. I studied Foot Zone Therapy with Charles in Norway and the United States and was certified by him in 1991. Charles, who died in 1995, was a very warm and kind man and powerful healer. He told us that he had been inspired through dreams about the proper dimensional placement for the body organs and systems in the feet. His visions were then transferred into numerous charts. The charts exemplified exquisite detail, particularly the charts featuring the great toe that focused on the vascular systems of the head and neck. [*See Figure 0-6*]

After studying with Charles and working with his charts, I came to politely refer to the majority of charts on the market in the United States as "kindergarten charts." These charts typically include only the major organs in general placement in the feet. Because they are so rudimentary, they are not really necessary. It is possible to identify the placement of the organs once one knows the basic structure of the hologram, which will be discussed later in this chapter. But when the hologram becomes more complicated, such as in certain areas and systems of the body like the pelvis and the lymphatic system with its diffuse network of vessels, nodes, ducts, and trunks, charts drawn by experienced foot reflexology and Foot Zone Therapy practitioners are helpful to those who are learning. Charles's charts are

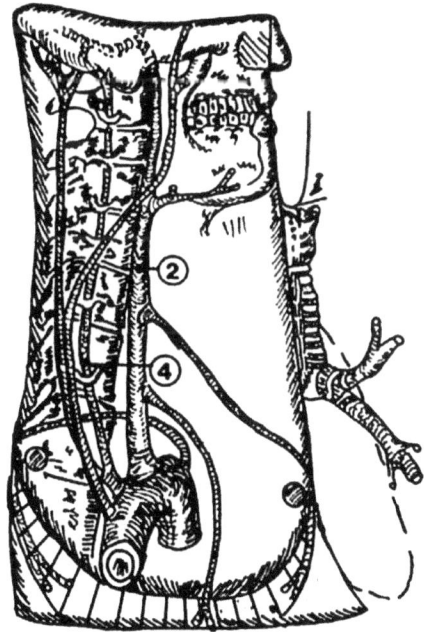

0-6 EXAMPLE OF A SECTION OF ERSDAL CHART

conclusive. I learned more about human anatomy and physiology in my study with Charles than I had in seven years of higher education in nursing and dance therapy.

Charles, a medical doctor and acupuncturist as well as a Foot Zone therapist, followed the scientific development in zone therapy techniques of American physician William FitzGerald (1872-1942) from the earlier twentieth century. FitzGerald, who referred to his work as "zone analgesia,"[1] and subsequent zone therapists such as Charles have not been definitive about the workings of zone therapy, the origin of which is akin to reflexology. But the early hypotheses of zone therapy were that prolonged massage to a particular tender reflex point caused a counterirritant (increased circulation) effect with its accompanying sympathetic healing reflex in the associated organ.[2] Zone therapists and reflexologists also work to open electrical channels related to the nerve endings in the reflexes of the feet by working out the crystalline deposits of uric acid that form on the nerve endings that block the free flow and grounding of energy through the feet to the earth. Another hypothesis of noted reflexologists Kevin and Barbara Kunz is that reflexology "works" when proprioceptive centers in the feet stimulate responses in the autonomic and sensorimotor nervous system.[3]

I have tested all of these theories in practice over the years and have concluded that they all hold some merit. There is an important physiological effect that occurs when the different points or energy fields for the organs and body systems are touched that relieves pain, stimulates the nervous system to attend to healing a specific organ or process in the body, and removes uric acid crystal buildup in the feet that occurs naturally in the course of moving through life in an upright

---

1   (FitzGerald & Bowers, 1917)
2   (FitzGerald & Bowers, 1917)
3   (Kunz & Kunz, 2013)

stance. But all of these hypotheses do not necessarily tap into the inner workings of this ancient healing modality of touching the feet in a purposeful way. The notion that it is possible to activate the hologram or tap into the blueprint of the body in a state of perfect wholeness by touching points on the feet does make sense in theory and in practice.

My first foot reflexology teacher, a German healer named Margarete Teuwen, known as Oma ("grandmother" in German), knew that the tradition she was passing to me was that of spiritual connection with the "divine blueprint" of wholeness through the feet. So when Charles, another reflexology/zone therapy expert, taught me years later that when we touched the foot we were sending not only a "signal" to the brain through the nerve endings in the feet but were also sending a signal to the "blueprint," my interest in the science was piqued further. I am a simple student of quantum physics and the relationship of holograms and the human body. Therefore, this is not a book about holographic science. It will, however, lead you to further reading and study should you, too, be smitten with the spirit of inquiry. What remains here is my knowledge and experience of what actually happens in SEF treatments—energetically, spiritually, and physically. It takes time for inductive and deductive processes to sync experience with knowledge. I do know well that this seemingly elusive science is accessible to those who think deeply about the body as the manifestation or temple for spirit or energy flow.

The blueprint for the wholeness as energy flow or spirit is like a seed within each person. Human beings possess that blueprint just as an oak tree retains the blueprint of its manifestation first as a tiny acorn. Some focus on the human blueprint as DNA; however, it is more than that. Here is how we can know this. Look in the mirror at the anatomical structures of your face and ask yourself, "If each of our body parts contain the exact same DNA, how does the nose *know* to become a nose and not an ear?" What is that process about? This is due to what is referred to as "the blueprint" in SEF. The blueprint is best discussed, if not understood, in terms of scientific ideas about holograms, memory, energy fields, and light. The evolution of our understanding of the blueprint in SEF draws upon the work of scientists, such as Rupert Sheldrake's writings on the science of memory and morphic fields[4] and David Bohm's classic book, **Wholeness and the Implicate Order.** In this book, Bohm defines the holomovement as the "carrier" of the implicate order[5] of the universe.[6] Holomovement is defined as "an unbroken and undivided totality."[7] He writes that:

> *The key feature of the functioning of the hologram, i.e., in each region of space, the order of a whole illuminated structure is "enfolded" and "carried" in the movement of light. Something similar happens with a signal that modulates a radio wave. In all cases, the content or meaning that is "enfolded" or "carried" is primarily an order and a measure, permitting the development of a structure ... with the hologram far more subtle structures can be involved in this way (notably three-dimensional structures, visible from many points of view)."[8]*

In the application and translation of this science to SEF as a healing art, the word "totality" holds similar meaning to understanding of the "entirety." Bohm's explanation of the holomovement becomes the rationale for the invocation, ablution, and all SEF techniques in which the purpose is to use the hands to remove blockages to energy flow by

---

4   (Pribram & Broadbent, 1970; Sheldrake, 1995)
5   The implicate order is a dimension of existence in which all events and things are enfolded in wholeness and unity. This is differentiated from the explicate order, which is a dimension of seemingly isolated events and things in space and time.
6   (Bohm, 1980, p. 191)
7   (Bohm, 1980, p. 191)
8   (Bohm, 1980, p. 190)

invoking light to activate flow according to the divine blueprint accessible through the hologram. Sheldrake defines a hologram as a "physical record of interference patterns in the electro-magnetic field"[9] in which each part holds within it the blueprint for replicating the whole. He also states that "fields are not material objects, but regions of influence."[10] In SEF, body organs and systems are referred to as energy fields so as to differentiate them from the physical organs and systems.

The reason that it is important to know that SEF works by accessing the blueprint is because this is what differentiates this healing modality from others, such as the practice of medicine. Whereas medicine and SEF involve the knowledge of anatomy and physiology, the focus of that effect is quite dissimilar. In SEF, the focus is sending a signal to the blueprint and activating a subsequent release of energy into the corresponding field represented as an organ or body system. The purpose is to move energy in that organ and system and allow the consciousness of the divine blueprint to dictate the change necessary to manifest healing. This may sound paranormal to some, but to those who experience SEF and those, such as indigenous healers, who experience activation of different states of consciousness to help others, this process is commonly understood.

The blueprint for the body in its perfect, healthy, and whole state is stored in a dimension beyond time and space that is accessible through a shift in consciousness beyond physical perception in this dimension of space and time. Even when a person is missing a body part as a result of surgery or an accident, that body part still exists in the dimension of the blueprint. Some scientists, such as Pribram and Bohm,[11] have deeply explored the possibility that the universe is a

---

9   (Sheldrake, 1995, p. 78)
10   (Sheldrake, 1995, p. 78)
11   (Bohm, 1980)

hologram providing a platform in the West for greater explanation of experiences dubbed "paranormal" because they defy current scientific framework for explanation. Holographic theory,[12] as represented in ancient wisdom teachings East and West, provides a platform for the possibility of a different reality with the brain at the holographic center. The holographic notion that what is "above" is represented in that which is "below" is foundational to ancient wisdom teachings East and West from Hinduism to Hermeticism.[13] And yet in the material plane, that which is below is illusion, just as the reflection of an image in a mirror is basically illusion.

Illusion is neither good nor bad. It is a challenging part of life, however—particularly for the scientist who seeks to differentiate the "real" from the "unreal." SEF is a healing work that seeks to access that which is beyond illusion-reality dualism. When looking squarely through the lens of understanding that the whole-person form is manifest in the structures of the feet, we begin to see as well as sense the presence of holographic projection. One example of a common experience of the hologram that people have during an SEF treatment is the response to the working of the sinus areas of the head. People typically experience a clearing or opening of the sinuses when the reflexes are worked. The sinuses may open and drain if they are blocked with mucous, and thought processes clear. Clear sinuses are vital to breathing, the process that nourishes all of our body systems and organs with energy or life force as well as oxygen. The basic SEF treatment, as discussed further in Chapter 1, includes the opening of the sinus energy fields.

All actions during SEF occur in the flow of energy through the points or energy fields in the feet that represent each organ or body

---

12   (Talbot, 1991)

13   (Hauck, 1999)

system. When we talk about an action in SEF, such as opening the sinus energy fields, we are referring only to the flow of energy. There is a difference between moving energy in the sinus energy fields by sending a signal to the blueprint and treating the sinuses as we might do in self-care like flushing out with salt water using a a Neti Pot or seeking the help of a physician who performs a medical or surgical procedure to open the sinus cavity. This may seem obvious, but I have found over the years that it is best to remind ourselves and anyone we may help with SEF that the specific focus of SEF is energy flow related to organs and systems, not the medical treatment of them. SEF moves energy or qi, thereby allowing for the wisdom of the body's natural processes to work more freely to establish and maintain balance, harmony, and health. The next key to SEF is to know how to identify the blocks within the energy fields of the hologram of the organs and body systems. Blocks are identified through placement, pain, and patterns.

Placement

Being able to recognize energy blockages comes with experience working with the hologram of the feet in which the energy is flowing through a specific organ or system field and ones in which the energy is not. Although a hologram of the entirety is also reflected in the hand and the ear, the hologram in the feet is much easier to learn and treat. The feet have clear landmarks regardless of size, making it easier to identify the *placement* of the organs and systems of the body. This is one of the major reasons that the focus of SEF and therefore this book is the hologram in the feet.

Learn the placement of body organs and body systems as they are scaled down in the feet first by looking at your feet as a whole. In SEF, both feet are a representation of the whole body in its entirety.

The right foot represents the right side of the body and the left foot represents the left side of the body. In the central nervous system, the left brain controls the right side of the body and vice versa. This function is taken into account in the practice of SEF, such as when working with stroke victims. The head of the human body is represented in the toe and the pelvis is represented in the heel. A major anatomical connection between the head and the pelvis is the spine. To locate the placement of the spine, sit in an upright seated position. If you are able, cross one of your feet over your knee so that you are now looking at the inner aspect of that foot. The human spine is in the midline of the body and is therefore located on the inner aspects of both feet. For this exercise, you can choose to work with either foot.

Rub your fingertips along the boney prominences along the inner side of your foot. [*See Figure 0-7*] Notice that they form a curved line from the flat inner side of the ankle area to the great toe. Next, rub your fingers on the back of your neck directly along the bony ridges of your cervical spine. Feel those bony prominences on the inner side of the foot again. They will feel very similar to the touch. Now move your fingers along the base of your neck. You should feel a slightly larger bump there. This is the cervical (C7) vertebra. Now turn your attention to the inner side of your foot. If you rub the area of the foot at the base of the great toe, you will notice that the C7 bump on the inner part of the foot feels very much like the bump on the back of the neck at the C7 vertebra! Move your fingers down the spine on your back until you reach the sacrum or flat bone at the base of the spine. Now move your fingers along the inner aspect of your foot. The hologram of the spine in the feet looks and feels like an actual spine. It also should be shaped

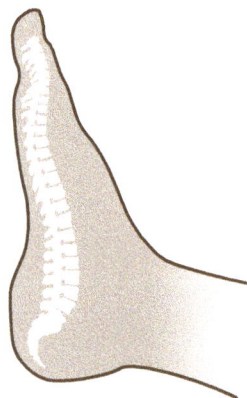

0-7 FOOT AND SPINE

like an "S" (on its side in the foot) with the vertebrae stacked like blocks. I have had clients who have had major car crashes in their lifetimes in which they sustained severe injuries to their spine. The residual injury from those crashes is often palpable in the hologram of the feet. SEF treatment of the energy blockages that occur as a result of those spinal injuries is possible. This will be discussed later in the book.

The head, pelvis, and spine are some of the most important placements to learn in the practice of SEF. But there are some more general placements or landmarks that are equally, if not more, fundamental to SEF work. The

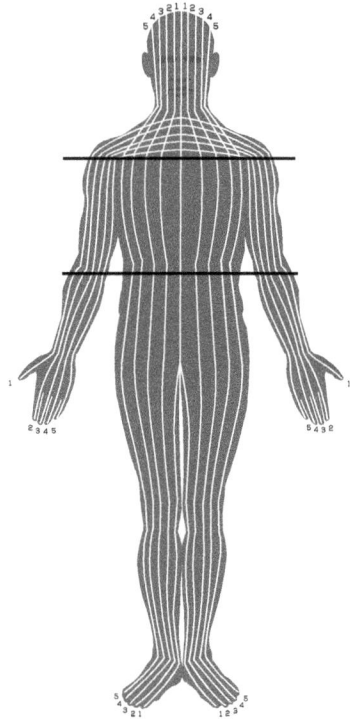

0-8 TEN ZONES

first of these placements has to do with the ten zones of the body. The midline of the body front and back represents the first zones. [*See Figure 0-8*] Moving laterally from the midline are zones two through five on the right and left. The thumbs and great toes are zone one and each toe and finger moving laterally are zones two through five. All organs and body systems within a particular zone are affected by changes within that zone. This energetic relationship between organs and systems within a zone will be discussed further in the section on "patterns."

The transverse zones are essential elements for use in the location of internal organs and body systems and structures. The transverse zones, or shoulder and waistlines, are drawn on the feet. [*See Figure 0-9*]. Remembering that the head area is represented in the toes, you will find that the shoulder line runs across the foot as it

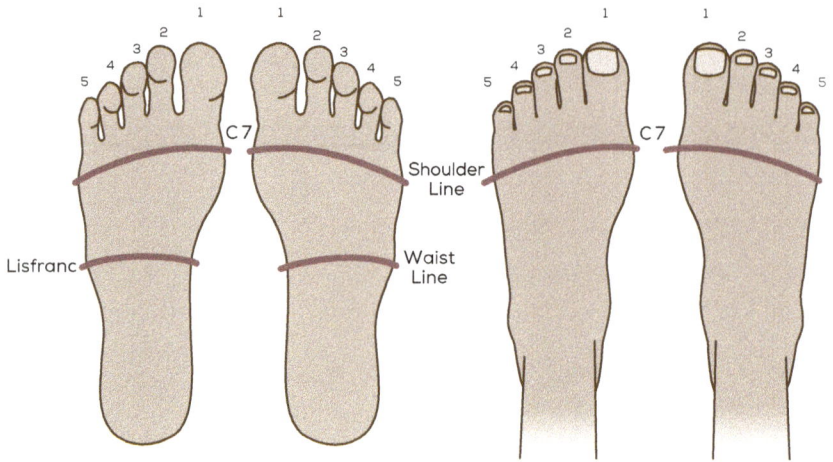

0-9   TRANSVERSE ZONES ON THE FEET

does in the body and includes the base of the neck (C7) as identified in the spine and foot illustration in zone one and the shoulder in zone five at the base of the small toe. If you touch the outer edge of the prominence at the base of the small toe and then touch the outer side of your shoulder, you will feel a similarity as you did with C7.

The waistline in any pair of feet is located first by touching the bony prominence in the fifth zone on the outer part of the Lisfranc joint complex (the midfoot). Then use your finger to trace a slightly arched line from the Lisfranc joint to the middle of the arch of the foot. This is the waistline that denotes the placement for all organs that lie between the shoulders and the waist. Examples of these organs are the liver and the spleen.

Figure 0-10 shows the vertical zones as they are scaled down in the feet. These zones also help when identifying the placement of organs within

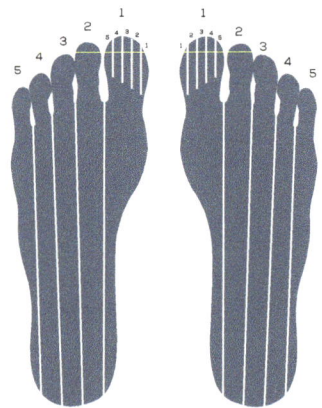

0-10   TEN ZONES ON THE FEET

the hologram of the feet. For example, a healthy thyroid gland is positioned in the throat at the midline of the body. It is shaped like a butterfly with two "wings" located in zone one. The gland does not extend past zone one. SEF treatment of the energy field for the thyroid gland includes working the area on the underside of the foot in a horizontal motion from the C7 area to the end of zone one between the great and second toes. How the thyroid or the field of any organ is worked with the hands will be covered in subsequent pages.

Pain

As discussed above, when first learning SEF, an organ is typically located in the hologram of the feet using landmarks and mental awareness of where a particular body part is in relationship to other structures, such as the shoulder or waistline, or the response of the person receiving SEF. Please note that in this book, the recipient of SEF will be referred to as the "Partner" and the person giving the SEF as the "Provider." The reason for this is to distinguish those who may not be licensed health professionals who provide SEF from licensed health professionals who typically refer to people they treat as "patients" or "clients." Feedback from the Partner of the SEF treatment is also important to confirm the placement of an energy field of an organ or system in the feet. Partners often experience pain when the fingers of the SEF Provider come in contact with a specific field. One clear example of this occurs when working the gallbladder (GB). The GB is a small pear-shaped sac located behind the liver. It receives bile from the liver through ducts or openings and then during digestion the walls of the GB contract to secrete bile into the small intestine (SI). The energy flow is moved in the hologram of the feet as it is naturally in the physiology of the body and so the hand actions of the SEF Provider mimic that flow. In order to assist the GB in contracting and secreting bile into the SI, the Provider must first locate the energy field of the GB itself. The GB is located in zone 3 to 4 of the right foot above the waistline and below the shoulder line. But the liver is also present in this area of the foot. Touching the GB in the foot requires a hand motion that lifts the field of the liver and reaches behind it. Contact with the GB may be experienced as pain but typically not until the proper action is made to connect with it behind the liver.

The pain that occurs when pressing a point on the feet is a signal to the brain that complements the SEF signal to the holographic blueprint. People most often report this pain that they experience as tolerable and hurting in a "good way." The pain should not be provoked for the sake of activating pain response as was done by early twentieth-century zone therapists. It is also not necessary to repeatedly stimulate the pain response in an energy field point on the feet. In SEF, it is only necessary to "ring the bell" and send the signal for that particular point once in a session. The pain that is sometimes experienced is also not typically sustained, though this can happen. Techniques for remedying such a reaction will be discussed in Chapters 1 and 3.

Pain experienced during SEF can be interpreted for the person as a "blockage of energy flow" in the field related to that body part. It should also be explained to a Partner that pain does not mean that there is something medically "wrong" with that part of the body. Some people are used to interpreting their pain only in biomedical diagnostic terms. In SEF, pain is related to an energetic pattern. Those who engage in SEF often need assistance in learning a new culture of health care that focuses on energy flow and health patterns.

Patterns

Any disruption in the body's equilibrium is reflected energetically in some way in the zones of the feet. SEF includes simple techniques for affecting and effecting that equilibrium by moving energy perceived as blockages in the energy field and recognized in the hologram of the feet. There are three ways that SEF Providers can recognize these blockages. First, by knowing the overarching blueprint that is "normal" to human anatomy and physiology really well, one can project that understanding onto the feet that are being treated and make comparisons between the energy field of the organ felt and the knowledge of what should be.

Second, the Provider gathers the health story of the person he or she is helping. The story typically represents the person's principal concerns. Over the years, I have found that people typically reveal the most important and relevant information about their health pattern at some point during an SEF session. In nursing and medicine, the practice of health history taking is often performed with the purpose of "assessing" or interrogating the person before giving any care because the treatment chosen is then based upon that assessment and subsequent diagnosis. The diagnosis is a synthesis statement of the analysis of a person's problems and/or needs given the findings of the assessment. In SEF, assessment, diagnosis, and care occur simultaneously. They actually occur simultaneously in nursing and medicine as well, but that is another story. In SEF, the focus is "reading" the health pattern in the story that the Partner tells and integrating that knowledge gained from the story with the energy patterns felt in the feet.

Health patterns are multidimensional because people are multidimensional. Therefore, the SEF Provider takes what a person expresses during their health story as a reference point for comparing the actual to the potential—what is felt in the energy fields of the feet to the blueprint represented in awareness of normal anatomy and physiology. What Oma taught me, and my observations confirm, is that no pair of feet feels or responds the same way from treatment to treatment. SEF is responsive to dynamic energy patterns in the feet that change frequently in relationship to internal and external stimuli. An SEF Provider processes all of this information consciously and unconsciously.

The third source of information that serves to create an understanding of the Partner's health pattern is the pattern of changes that occur in the various organs and systems over time. These changes are noticed with the senses. The SEF Provider may actually see certain places on the feet respond differently. A common example is that certain points light up or turn red and may remain so for a period of time. The Provider may hear the Partner express pain as discussed above and may also feel changes such as muscle contractions through a developed sense of touch.

The SEF Provider attunes to or locates organs and body systems as energy fields in the feet through touch. As the hands and fingers move around the feet, there are detectable changes in energetic patterns. While some of these changes one perceives are more general to the entirety, some of the energy changes felt are subtler. These felt energy changes can be perceived as the shape of the body organs. For example, the human kidney is shaped somewhat like a kidney bean. The energy field of the kidney in the foot has subtle definition that is actually bean shaped.

These energy patterns co-exist and, therefore, time and experience in working peoples' feet really helps with detection, discernment, and interpretation of the various energy patterns using touch and kinesthetic senses. Our kinesthetic sense is related to proprioception, which is the ability to perceive the body's position in space and the effort employed in movement. Training the kinesthetic sense and touch is possible. One of the first experiences that helped me most in sensing organ energy patterns in the feet kinesthetically and through touch occurred during my one-to-one training with an experienced nurse at Children's Hospital in Los Angeles in 1986. I was a new graduate nurse on an infant specialty care unit. My mentor gave me a tremendous learning experience in pattern recognition when I needed to start intravenous (IV) lines in babies' veins. She turned off the lights and, rather than use my eyes to look for the vein, she made me feel for the chubby babies' veins by sensing movement of blood flow. The accuracy with which we were able to get the intravenous (IV) lines placed in tiny babies' veins with one needle stick really amazed me. She taught me the power of trusting the ability to assess through touch and my sense of movement. Veins are palpable and so are energy fields in the hologram of the feet! The first step to recognizing those fields is to know human anatomy and physiology and then train ones' kinesthetic sense and sense of touch. I still close my eyes and work in a dimly lit room when offering SEF in order to engage my senses more deeply so that I can better perceive and locate the energy fields of organs in the feet.

SEF draws upon knowledge of the science of pattern recognition utilized in the health professions, such as nursing and Traditional Chinese Medicine. It also employs knowledge of energetic patterns represented in the sciences of human anatomy, physiology, kinesiology (the study of movement) and ideo-kinesiology (the study of imagery and movement). Working with people's feet leads to greater understanding of their life story and the life path they have walked. American reflexologist Eunice Ingham (1889-1974) wrote two classic books called *Stories the Feet Can Tell* (1938) and *Stories the Feet Have Told* (1963). SEF incorporates knowledge from these early writings by Ingham[14] and FitzGerald with my education and training with Oma and Charles in foot reflexology and zone therapy, and some of the clinical research that has been conducted. It also extends their works through the integration of healing traditions, such as the application of topical plant remedies, and attention to health pattern recognition, which provides keys to the nature of the soul (aka the sole of the foot) in the effort to bring about greater harmony, balance, and comfort as a person walks their life path.

Bohm, D. (1980). *Wholeness and the Implicate Order*. London: Routledge Classics.

FitzGerald, W., & Bowers, E. (1917). *Zone Therapy*. Columbus, Ohio: I.W. Long.

Hauck, D. (1999). *The Emerald Tablet*. New York: Penguin Group.

Kunz, B. & Kunz, K. (2013). Reflexology Research. 2013, from http://www.reflexology-research.com

Pribram, K., & Broadbent, D. (1970). *Biology of Memory*. New York: Academic Press.

Sheldrake, R. (1995). *The Presence of the Past: Morphic Resonance and the Habits of Nature*. Rochester, Vermont: Park Street Press.

Talbot, M. (1991). *The Holographic Universe*. New York: Harper Perennial.

---

14   Dwight Byers and his sister, a nurse named Eusebia Messenger, continued the work of their aunt Eunice Ingham upon her death in 1974. Byers and his wife, Nancy, are the founders of the International Institute of Reflexology®

CHAPTER ONE

◌

Preparation for the Basic SEF Treatment

Foot reflexology is practiced all over the world. While in some cultures, "working the feet" may be part of a standard of care in the dominant health care system, the practice is found primarily in clinics, private offices, spas, and "boutique" health centers. For many years, I have offered SEF to clients in my private holistic nursing practice as a modality—and I still do. However, for the past 10 years, it has become an integral part of my assessment and care for all clients. I realized that I had come to rely on the information I had received about the clients' health patterns from the feet and that my care was, in fact, more holistic when I accessed the hologram of the feet. Anecdotally, I had also observed that clients progressed more quickly when receiving SEF treatments as part of care. I had returned to a practice similar to what I had in the 1990s while providing holistic nursing care to people in a rural community in the northwestern United States where biomedical practitioners were scarce.

SEF is one of, if not *the*, most accessible, affordable, effective, and holistic treatments on the planet today. After more than three decades of helping people both with and without SEF, I have come to the realization that the ancestors got it right! Working the feet, our "under-standing," is simply foundational to self-care and health care in which we truly seek to promote healing. It is easily accessible in that the instruments of care for self or others are the hands we have with us at all times. There is no expensive technology (equipment or drugs), although time is one commodity involved in an SEF treatment. It can be provided to oneself or it can be offered to another free of charge as a gesture of loving service. It can also be a part of a community's health care system if it is structured in such a way as to support lay Providers and professional practitioners with the time they need to render SEF as part of caring services. Comparative research on health care services may ultimately show someday that inclusion of SEF in care is ultimately more affordable and more cost effective than trying to provide care without the insight gained as a result of SEF treatment.

There are three phases of an SEF basic treatment: Preparation, Initiation, and Sealing. Chapters 2 and 3 deal with the initiation phase and Chapter 4 the sealing. This chapter deals with the 4 A's of preparation: attunement, ablution, anointing, and approach.

Preparation begins with setting intention. If that intention is first and foremost to make money or derive personal power over another, a Provider may find that full "access"[1] to the divine blueprint and understanding of health patterns may be limited or denied. Consider the ancient maxim recorded biblically as, "But seek ye first the kingdom of God, and his righteousness; and all these things shall be added unto you."[2] In SEF, "seeking God" can be interpreted as setting an intention to pursue an understanding of the Creator as manifest in Self and others through kindness and service. This intention is central

---

1   By this, I refer to a mystical quotient in which one's vibration in consciousness, as attainment through spiritual preparation, contains a code to releasing understanding as a key is coded and patterned by a locksmith to open a lock.
2   (Bible, 1972, Matthew 6:33)

to the effectiveness of SEF as a holistic treatment—that which heals spirit, mind, and emotion as well as body. Preparation for providing a basic SEF treatment first includes a practice of attunement with the flow of spirit in service to humanity.

ATTUNEMENT

SEF should not be reserved only for those who can pay boutique fees. It is also not a poor man's medicine used in self-care by default because that person cannot afford the best in biomedical treatments. It is important to preserve the integrity of healing traditions such as SEF and recognize the potential for the vibration of a materialistic culture to penetrate our beliefs, practices, and systems of health care in ideas such as these. SEF can actually be offered to anyone in any venue. I have treated people—from world leaders to criminals and newborns to centenarians—in their homes, offices, clinics, and hospitals; by the pool, stream, or ocean; and in hotel rooms, cars, and airplanes. The integrity of this tradition is sustained first through the consciousness of the SEF Providers as they attune to the flow of spiritual essence and living ethic of care that is SEF. Renowned psychologist and researcher of optimal experience, Dr. Mihaly Csikszentmihalyi, writes:

> Flow helps to integrate the self because in that state of deep concentration consciousness is unusually well ordered. Thoughts, intentions, feelings and all the senses are focused on the same goal. Experience is in harmony. And when the flow episode is over, one feels more "together" than before, not only internally but also with respect to other people and to the world in general.[3]

---

3   (Csikszentmihalyi, 1990, p. 41)

In SEF, the Provider enters a state of consciousness of meditation or complete disciplined concentration on the energy flow in the feet, visualizing the blueprint of wholeness manifest in the hologram of anatomy and physiology, and the feedback that comes through in the Partner's responses to care.

In this state of attunement and flow, there is no need to think or reflect with the mind because "the action carries us forward as if by magic."[4] As the SEF Provider accesses this state of consciousness during treatment, the energy is conveyed to the Partner. I like to refer to this attunement practice as "holding the balance." I use the image of the pre-digital scales of Lady Justice for this. As the Provider enters the state of attunement with the Partner, the two come into balance with each other. The Provider enters the world of the SEF Partner to perform the healing work. Holding the balance becomes especially important when someone is in a state of crisis or major transition such as birth or death.

It is during attunement that the Provider prepares oneself to enter the world of the Partner. Because people often seek healing at times when they are in crisis, it is important for the Provider who would enter the world of the Partner to know how to maintain one's boundaries or protect oneself spiritually so as not to become confused that the energetic patterns of another are one's own. Spiritual protection was not really something I learned about in nursing school even though some very spiritual people educated me. I was simply taught to "pray." However, the spiritual teaching on protection as a practitioner handed down to me from Oma is much more active.

The potential for change and healing as an activation and increase of energy flow or light in the body from an SEF treatment is

---

4   (Csikszentmihalyi, 1990, p. 54)

profound. However, the level of flow and, therefore, light released is directly proportional to the momentum of preparation and attunement as well as the level of protection that the Providers are able to invoke as they create the environment in which they hold the balance for the release of flow and light. This is an innate protection within the healing tradition of SEF that is particularly important for the novice Provider to realize.

Many ask me if they can "hurt" someone by giving an SEF treatment. If the spiritual as well as physical steps presented in this book are followed, then the risk of "hurting" another is similar to the risk undertaken when cooking them a meal or driving them in your car to an appointment. The SEF Provider is kindly extending the hand of caring compassion to help and heal. If these spiritual tenets of the tradition are not followed, then the power of the SEF treatment is significantly diminished to the mundane—that of offering a relaxing foot rub.

Attunement is the first step in preparing to provide a basic SEF treatment that is much more than a foot rub. There is nothing wrong with a foot rub! My husband knows I love them. I cannot count the number I have had from him in 20 years. But there are also many times when the foot rub has not been enough to move the energy needed to create the change that can lead to healing.

The quality of an SEF treatment, whether done at home in self or family care or at a professional clinic, is different from a foot rub. It is also completely different from a massage. There are some motions used in SEF, which will be discussed later, in which massage techniques are used to move energy in the entirety of the feet. However, attunement rituals applied by the Provider are the first step in setting a different tone for care to be given that defines SEF treatment.

There are some physical preparations that the Provider needs to do prior to providing an SEF treatment. First, fingernails must be cut and filed so that they are very short and soft without jagged or sharp edges or borders. After cutting the nails, take an emery board and file the corners of the nails to ensure that the edges are rounded and smooth. This is of particular importance with the thumbnails. Then file each nail over the top of the edge toward the finger so as to soften the edge of the nail.

It is a requirement to trim the nails because nails of the Provider can cause pain and damage to the skin of the Partner's feet. Because this pain is not related to the release of energy in the hologram but a physical response to a stimulus, the Provider can make an incorrect assumption of the pattern. The ritual of cutting the nails is the first "test" of willingness to serve others. Over the years, I have had a number of women enter my SEF classes having just had expensive manicures and "tips" put on their nails. They realize often more quickly than other students that offering SEF requires some planning ahead and changes in health and beauty habits. SEF can also be very physically challenging. Providers offer their bodies as instruments of healing service to another. Therefore, the Providers attune their own bodies to the energy involved in the work through physical exercise, proper rest, nourishment through food and play, and intimacy with others and God, the Creator. I find dance to be one form of physical preparation that is most congruent with SEF attunement. This may be because dance, and all movement actually, can be described in scientific terms related to effort or exertion patterns defined as weight, time, space, and *flow*.

Flow in movement science relates to the degree of tension in a movement on a quality scale from "free" to "bound," with bound flow being more tense and free flow more relaxed. Neither bound nor free flow is better than the other. However, the appropriateness of a behavioral response from the perspective of effort/flow can be interpreted when taken in context. Extreme bound or restricted flow is appropriate flow of energy when carrying a pot of hot coffee from the kitchen to the dining room whereas applying the energy pattern of a bull in the china shop would not be appropriate.

Changes in flow occur throughout the body all day long or at least they should. The body's ability to shift in effort/flow from free to bound allows a person to respond to environmental stimuli. One of the reasons SEF is helpful to people is that the treatment period acts as a re-set of the body's responses. People often seek treatment when they are under extreme stress. The body and the hologram in the feet will typically demonstrate the effect of the extreme stress and subsequent excess state of bound flow. These effects will be explored in a later chapter after explaining basic treatment practices in more detail.

Take a moment now and attune to your own body. Start at the top of your head and imagine that you are drawing light and energy from the sun into your head. In this exercise of preparation and attunement, just focus on allowing the light to move all stagnant qi patterns in larger regions of the body rather than focusing on organs. As the light moves into the head region, imagine those energy blocks, which may feel like tension, as darkened. Allow the light to penetrate those areas and disperse the darkness and, with it, the tension. During the body attunement exercise, you may want to tense and release muscles, such as the muscles of the face or the abdomen or buttocks as you imagine the light displacing or illuminating the dark blockages.

Just as musicians tune their instruments before playing, SEF Providers tune their body instruments through attunement exercises such as this. Just as musicians tune up so that they play the right notes and the sound they make is the right pitch, Providers prepare their body and hands, in particular, to receive and send energy and clear signals unimpeded by their personal stressors, emotional concerns, distracting thoughts, and spiritual distress. All of these personal challenges can be set aside for a period of time as you focus your attunement and attention on serving another person with SEF.

ABLUTION

Albert Einstein is quoted as having said, "The most beautiful and most profound emotion we can experience is the sensation of the mystical." One can feel the sensation of the mystical in the preparation for an SEF treatment—particularly the second phase, which is during the ritual of the washing of the feet. Oma taught me her way of applying this ancient practice used by Jesus and other healers throughout the centuries in modern-day foot reflexology practice. The ritual includes an herbal footbath and the use of the hands to strip the energy fields of the feet, a practice I refer to as "ablution." An ablution is the term for ritual washing for the purpose of purification. Ablution is found in many cultures, including Islamic (Wudu - partial ablution as opposed to full-body ablution), Judaism, Shinto (Misogi), and Christian[5] traditions.

There is evidence for the positive physical, emotional, mental, and spiritual effects of footbaths. For example, there are numerous articles published on the positive effects of hot footbaths on sleep.[6] The history of Christianity includes evidence that the spiritual meaning of the ritual of the washing of the feet exemplified by Jesus the Christ when he washed the disciples' feet[7] was spiritual cleansing, forgiveness, and preparation to enter the presence of God.[8] One scholar concluded that the Johannine community continued the tradition

---

5   (Bible, 1972, John:13)

6   (Liao, Landis, Lentz, & Chiu, 2005; Sung & Tochihara, 2000)

7   (Bible, 1972, John:13)

8   (Knox, 1950)

after Jesus' death, but that the cleansing produced by the act had "eschatological" rather than ceremonial or sacramental meaning.[9] This means that the ritual realized the perfection of God's creation, the end of ordinary reality, and offered reunion with the Divine.

Purification and curing by water, particularly in psychiatry dating back to the centuries when water bathing was used to dispel evil spirits that possessed people's minds,[10] has been present in cultures across the globe for centuries, if not millennia. In my historical research, I have found footbaths to be a healing tradition in European and American nursing practices dating nearly 400 years.[11] Whether nurses acknowledge the religious history of foot bathing or its spiritual effects in their practice or not, footbaths remain a powerful instrument of healing in nurses' care and comfort for the physical, emotional, and psychological selves of patients. They can also be performed by anyone and are an essential element of preparation for SEF treatment. I will also add here that it is my observation that during the preparatory footbath before the basic treatment begins, the SEF Partner experiences healing as powerful energy flow. I attribute this to the historical momentum of the energy of healing that the footbath carries within the memory of peoples across the globe.

Despite the potential benefits of footbaths, reflexologists, for the most part, shun the idea of baths or any other topical applications to the feet for a variety of reasons. In SEF tradition, however, footbaths, herbal wraps, and anointing the feet with specially chosen medicinal-grade essential oils are all elements of that which makes

---

9   (Weiss, 1979, p. 325)
10   (Diamandopoulos, Vlachos, & Marketos, 1997, p. 26)
11   (Libster & McNeil, 2009, pp. 199-200)

a foot treatment distinctly SEF. Additional details of the herbal topical applications will be addressed in more detail in Chapter 4: *Sealing of the Feet and Herbal Stress Relief.*

Gather the supplies for the footbath and ablution. You will need:

1. Foot Bath Basin. For this, I suggest that you get a recyclable plastic basin typically sold as a "dishpan." The dimensions of the bottom of the basin are approximately 12x10 inches by 4 to 5 inches high. [*See Figure 1-1*] You can use the electric footbaths that vibrate and produce heat, but remember that this will change the energy field of the feet significantly. I do not use these in my practice for a number of reasons including the fact that the design of the upper collar makes it difficult to perform the ablution on larger feet and legs. Be sure to disinfect the basins after a footbath. Scrub the basin with hot soapy water using a dedicated brush, sponge, or washcloth. Rinse with warm water and then rinse with a cold bleach water solution as per your household cleaning guidelines or per local public health guidelines if you are a professional practitioner.

2. One cotton bath towel. Use cotton towels, as they are absorbent.

3. Two cotton hand towels. These should be thin rather than plush as they will be used to wrap the feet later on; plush towels are harder to stretch and tuck around the foot.

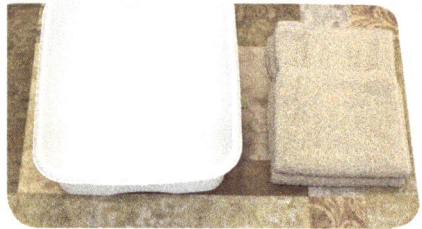

1-1 FOOTBATH SETUP

4. Herbal bath infusion, oil, salt etc. (Discussed in Chapter 4)

5. Comfortable chair for the Partner to sit in that supports a straight spine.

6. Light blanket for the Partner's shoulders if they are feeling cold.

Before putting your Partner's feet in a footbath, have them take off their shoes and socks or hose and roll up their pant legs above the mid-calf area. Be sure to inspect both feet for injury, wounds, and open sores that, if touched, might cause physical discomfort. Be sure to ask the Partner about any bruises, cuts, structural distortions, or damaged toenails you observe. You can also best hold the balance for your Partner if you first assess their perception of their own feet and what health challenges they are dealing with at the time.

Next, choose the remedies to include in the footbath. Details of the choices are discussed later but the general principle is to be sure to engage the Partner in the choice of footbath remedy. Plain water is healing, too, but the reason for considering a remedy during a footbath has to do, once again, with anatomy and physiology. Many people do not realize that some of the largest pores in the skin of the human body are found in the soles of the feet. During a warm footbath, those pores open and are able to readily absorb the healing effects of herbal and other remedies through the feet.

When I was training with Oma, she taught me about the pores in the feet with a really fun example. I was observing her while she was treating a client.[12] He was reclining in her special wooden reflexology chair, which allowed clients to be comfortably laid back with their feet up toward the ceiling so that we, the practitioners, could stand up to

---

12   In a professional SEF practice, a healing relationship is referred to as being between a practitioner and a client or patient; whereas, for the lay person providing SEF, the healing relationship is between the Provider and the Partner.

treat the feet. The position in the chair made the clients very relaxed. This client was very quiet and restful after his footbath. We moved him to the reflexology chair, covered him in a sheet, and laid him back. In demonstration of the nature of the pores in the soles of the feet, Oma put a single drop of dill essential oil on the bottom of one of his feet. He quietly mumbled, "Gee, my mouth is watering—are there a lot of dill pickles in here?" I could barely smell the drop that Oma had placed on his foot. His nose was a good distance from his feet too. He said that he actually tasted the dill. Because of the size of the pores, especially after a hot footbath, his experience of that single drop of dill oil was profound. Be very mindful that the choice of remedy in the footbath well suits the senses of your Partner!

Fill the basin two-thirds full. Follow hydrotherapy principles and make sure that the temperature of the water is hot enough (approximately 92 degrees F/33 degrees C) to produce a relaxation response. In the summer, I often use cool footbaths for people when their feet are hot, sore, and swollen from walking in the heat. Many people work in air conditioning and, therefore, more often have very cold feet even in summer, so the hot footbath is used year round. I do not use a thermometer anymore when testing the temperature of the footbath, but you may want to do so until you have the body memory of what it feels like on your body. Do not test the temperature of the footbath water with your hands, as they are often cold to begin with. Use your wrist or elbow. There have been many times that I have had to heat water on a stove or hotpot to add to the bath when treating people in facilities where the hot-water temperature is kept low so that people who use the facilities do not burn themselves.

When you present the basin to your Partner, put it in front of them on a bath towel the long way as shown in the picture. [*See Figure 1-1*] People's feet are longer than they are wide and therefore fit more comfortably in the basin placed in the long direction. Fold two hand towels in half the long way and then in half again and position them on the bath towel next to the basin with the folded edge toward you. Have your towels ready to use quickly after the feet have been in the bath so as to retain the warmth of the feet. I then put the bath remedy into the basin in front of the Partner and then swirl the water with my hand to check the temperature one last time and gently mix the remedy into the water using a figure eight swirling hand motion. This pattern reflects the same water motion found in nature in which water is purified.[13] Be mindful that you do not keep your own hands in the footbath water so long as to make it *your* bath water—energetically speaking. The footbath is the Partner's bath and will engage his/her energy and also draw out their body's "toxins." Try not to leave your mark. Just mix the remedy and water, then present the basin to the Partner and ask them to place their feet in it. After they confirm that the temperature is warm but not too hot, allow them to soak quietly. Ask them to meditate, pray, or center during the footbath while you do the same.

All three practices encourage connection with the Creator by any name— God, Yahweh, Allah, or the creative force of the universe. I have also treated atheists who connect with the force of healing energy in the universe, for example. Centering is a process of establishing a sense of balance in one's body while connecting with the Creator of the blueprint. Here is an exercise you can do to get a sense of what centering is in your body. Stand with your feet slightly apart below your shoulders with your arms by your side. This is called "place" in dance.

Place is considered to be a position of strength and balance. Bend to one side as far as you can go without moving your feet. Then come back to place. Observe how far you can bend without toppling over.

---

13 (Alexandersson, 1997)

Always come back to place and observe how easy or difficult it is on any given day. Pay attention to where place is when you find that stance or mark after bending to the side. That is your "center" or place of balance. Centering exercises promote a shift in consciousness and emotion, as well as physical sensation, back to a point of balance and strength. The more centering is practiced, the easier it becomes to know what takes one from the strength of center and what is needed to return to it. Ablution helps with establishing and maintaining a sense of place and balance. While the Partner's feet are in the water, I often leave the room for a few minutes while they enjoy the footbath alone so that they can bring their own centering practice to the footbath experience should they choose to do so.

I have learned in books and classes on hydrotherapy that, technically, the pores in the feet take at least 15 minutes to open. But in my practice I do a five- to 10-minute footbath with excellent results—and Oma did too. The ideal, however, is to keep the footbath warm for about 15 minutes to allow the pores to fully open. Try a footbath for yourself! It is a wonderful self-care remedy.

After the feet have soaked, kneel on the floor directly in front of the Partner. Take a moment for quiet centering. I like to look up into the face of the Partner and smile, acknowledging the beauty of their soul/sole. I then place the palm of my left hand on the instep of their right foot and my right hand on the instep of their left foot. The palms of your hands fully engage the top of the feet where you may feel the radiation of significant energy centers. Engaging the foot means connecting skin surface to skin surface and energy center to energy center. In this case, the energy centers or chakras in the hands engage the chakras in the feet while in the water for a powerful energetic bond.

While in this position, begin your protection visualizations, which allow you to stay energetically on "your side of the fence."

That is, you must maintain your personal boundaries and allow your Partner, who is now more vulnerable after having accepted the treatment, to do so also. A visualization for protection used in SEF is a lighthouse. Imagine yourself as a lighthouse all lit up in the night. Oma used to say with a chuckle that the darkness never enters the lighthouse, but the light spills out into the darkness of the night. When we visualize ourselves as a lighthouse full of light, it spills over to the Partner in need; any darkness or energy that would not necessarily be helpful to us or them that may come about as a result of SEF will, in this case, enter the footbath water and not our hands and arms. Imagine your hands covered with brilliantly white gloves so that when you touch your Partner, they will come in contact only with pure light energy that can be used for healing and comfort.

Keeping your hands on the feet, make an invocation using the power of the voice and throat chakra to charge the footbath and herbal remedy with light. One example of a simple invocation is, "Let there be light!" You can also ask the Partner if they would like to speak an invocation for their own healing. After the invocation and visualizations, you will do the ablution by stripping the energy fields of the feet. Visualize your white-gloved hands like swords that you use in cutting away any energy debris from the feet of your Partner that is not their own and, therefore, not beneficial for them.

Cup your hands and bring some of the water up over the ankle, bathing one leg. Encircle the lower leg with both hands, thumbs toward you with your palms and fingers holding the leg firmly. When working with smaller legs, your fingers and thumbs may cross. Keeping the palms and all fingers in contact with the leg, move your hands down the lower leg from calf to foot as you strip the energy out through and between the toes. Splash the water up the leg again and then strip the energy fields of the leg, ankle, foot, and toes again.

This stripping action is the ablution. The action should be intentional, firm, and quick without dragging or pinching the skin. Your effort is directed specifically at stripping the energy field of any negative energy that the feet have picked up simply from walking the Earth that could be harmful or debilitating to the Partner. The ablution is not a water massage or a washing of the feet in the sense of bathing. It is a spiritual and energetic action. For further study of body energy related to the field around the feet, I suggest studying books, such as *The Body Electric*.[14]

The major energy centers or chakras in the body are associated with the major endocrine glands. (See Chapter 2) When providing the ablution to the feet, you are also able to strip the glands/chakras of debris. You do not need to know in your outer consciousness what this debris or negative energy is or what it looks like. Just know that the common response of those who experience a footbath and ablution is that their feet "feel lighter" and "happier" when they are rid of the weight of negative energy.

Oma called this negative energy "effluvia," which is typically defined as "waste." She knew it as more than simple waste and had a terrific explanation by means of a story. When stripping the feet of effluvia from lower legs to toes, some of the energy you have stripped off will enter the water. You can also shake the energy that has now attached to your hands into the ground so that it is not put back into the bath water or on the feet. Oma taught me to visualize the energy entering the ground with violet light to transmute any potentially disruptive or harmful effects. She always told the story about why she discarded the footbath water down the toilet. Now I tell it.

---

14   (Becker & Selden, 1998)

In her early practice days, Oma was working in her clinic in Glendale, California, and there was a drought. She did not want to waste any water that might be reused so she thought that she would throw her used footbath water into the garden—that is, until she saw what grew up where she routinely threw the water. Large gnarly plants and roots grew that were pretty scary looking. She realized that it was the effluvia in the bath water that had affected the growth of the plants. This is why we make it a practice to send the footbath water down the toilet right after we wrap the feet following the footbath and ablution.

Wrapping the feet in the hand towels is the last part of the ritual. Take the first hand towel and open it horizontally. Offer it to your Partner with your open palms facing upward. This gesture of love and compassion depicted in so many paintings is referred to by Dr. John Diamond as the "Madonna gesture"; it is one that exemplifies the love of Mother that opens the heart and strengthens the thymus gland of the giver and the receiver.[15] You then receive each foot as a mother would her newborn infant, with tender care and awe. I am always in awe of the energetic effects of the ritual of the washing of the feet. People's faces change in minutes, becoming softer and more radiant as they let go of effluvia and manifest the light that replenishes their energy field and body.

Jesus must have understood the mystical healing ritual of the washing of the feet as a spiritual cleansing. The purpose of the SEF ritual is not simply to bathe the feet before treatment because they may be dirty. Partners often apologize for the state of their feet when they prepare to experience the washing of the feet during their first SEF treatment. They often think that we are cleaning the feet so that

---

15   (Diamond, 1979, p. 49)

we can touch them. But the SEF Provider who is fully focused on the energetic action of ablution will find that some of the cleanest feet are some of the most effluvia- or entity-ridden and some of the grubbiest feet the purest. Take, for example, sweet children who have been playing outside in a mud puddle during a summer rain.

The ritual is also peace-making. The simple act of kneeling before someone else and washing his or her feet demonstrates kindness and can create peace. It is very hard for a person to remain angry with someone who is washing his or her feet. Oma used to talk about this during her public demonstrations. People would smile when she recommended it for married couples. We also recommend that children wash their parents' feet. Children love to help their parents when there is illness or tension in the family and are often at a loss as to what they can contribute. In their pure-heartedness, children often provide tremendous healing when they perform the ritual of the washing of the feet.

Be sure to wrap each foot with a towel quickly and snugly to preserve the warmth from the footbath. Covering the feet also contains the energy field around the foot. The foot is best wrapped by first pulling one side of the towel over and around, then tucking in the flap over the toes, and then stretching and pulling the other side of the towel around the foot while holding the towel in place with the other hand. The last corner of the towel is secured by tucking it in at the ankle. You then place both of your Partner's feet squarely on the floor beside the basin. Then firmly push the tops of your Partner's feet with your palms. This is a very important part of the treatment in which you establish with the Partner that you are going to handle the energy/effluvia for a few minutes so that they can focus on receiving healing. It is also an action that makes a connection between the Partner's feet and Earth, which absorbs the effluvia we send away to it so that the feet can be charged with life-sustaining energy from the planet.

The towel wrap should be secure enough so that the Partner can walk slowly in the towel. If they are seated in a straight-backed chair, I then have them walk a few steps in the towels to get onto a table to lie down for treatment. The feet can also be treated one by one while holding them in your lap if the Partner is seated in a recliner. I often use this positioning for the elderly or anyone who cannot easily climb up onto a table. In the recliner, it is best to put pillows behind their back during the foot washing so that they can sit straighter as the first light is invoked. Then remove the pillows and help the Partner recline for the next part of the preparation—the anointing of the feet.

ANOINTING

After the ablution, be very mindful that your Partner and their feet are vulnerable until you finish the treatment and they put their socks and shoes back on. The person is very relaxed and closes their eyes because they trust you physically and energetically to provide a safe place for them to take part in their healing work. You are the one who now is to control the energy in the healing space on behalf of your Partner. You do this by keeping the feet covered when they are not being worked. Touching the feet mindfully and respectfully also does this. There are many ways to demonstrate mindfulness and respect in addition to keeping the feet covered. For example, it is also respectful to not touch the feet unless necessary. In SEF, the hands touch in a highly purposeful and deliberate way so as to send clear signals. Be mindful that you need only "ring the bell" for a particular point to send a signal (as discussed in the Introduction) and do not need to continue to work it over and over.

After the Partner is situated on the table or recliner, position them for comfort. The feet should be higher than the rest of the body when on a table. In addition to pillows for your Partner's head, you

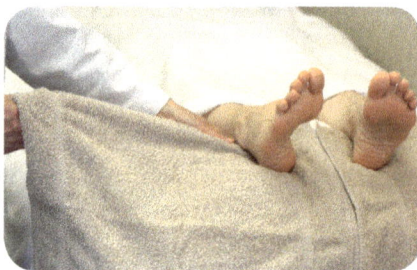

1-2 SEF TABLE SETUP

will also need to place a strong pillow or wedge under their knees and two to three pillows under their feet so that their feet are elevated. [*See Figure 1-2*] Cover the pillows with a sheet and the foot of the table with a bath towel for use later in the treatment. Once the person is on the table, open the foot towels and position them with the inner seams together between the feet. The rest of the towel will extend away from the foot and can be used to cover the foot when it is not being worked.

Next, you will use medicinal-grade eucalyptus essential oil to bridge the action of the ablution to the next step of preparation—anointing. The first time that you treat someone with any essential oil used neat or in an oil blend, be sure to have them sniff the bottle that you plan to use before applying the oil to your hands or their feet. If they have any negative reaction of any kind, do not use the oil. Essential and infused oil applications will be discussed further in Chapter 4. Place one drop of pure, medicinal-grade eucalyptus essential oil in each palm. Rub your hands together lightly and then, while visualizing your hands again as swords of light, use a quick, strong, direct hand action to strip the energy field of the lower legs and feet toward and out the toes a second time . You will notice that this oil is extremely etheric—that is, it dissipates rapidly into the atmosphere and leaves no residue on the skin. The purpose for its use in ablution is to strip away effluvia rather than to moisten the skin or deeply massage the tissues of the feet and legs. Work quickly so that you do not absorb all of the delicate molecules of the eucalyptus oil into your own skin and have nothing left for your Partner.

After the stripping action, shake any negative energy that you may have absorbed from your Partner's feet into the floor and visualize violet light or fire [*See Figure 1-3*] accompanying the energy into the Earth. This transferred energy may feel in your fingers, hands, or arms like needles poking you, pain, throbbing, stiffness, twisting or heaviness, to name a few

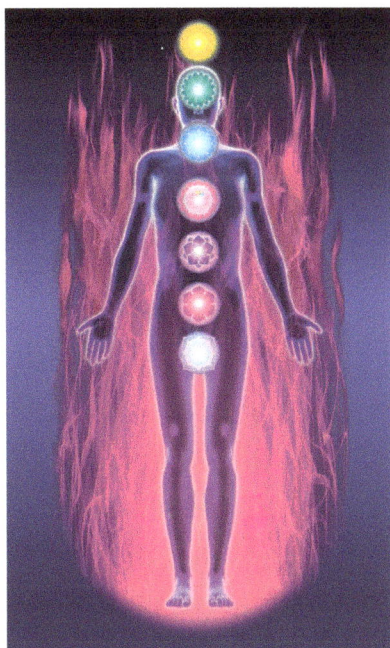

1-3   VIOLET FIRE

reactions. Never allow the negative energy from your Partner to creep up your arms to the elbows. You must protect your own health as energy flow by being mindful of if and when you have taken on energy through your hands and arms. Stop and shake it off while you visualize transmuting the energy with violet fire. Do not engage the energy emotionally, such as allowing yourself to express feelings of fear, anger, or disgust. Shake it off in a matter-of-fact way; redirect your focus to something of beauty, and continue on.

Cover the feet with the hand towels. You are now ready to begin the anointing with specially prepared massage oil. Take your chosen massage oil and pour a small amount into your hand. I like to use a glass dropper in my bottles so that I use only a squirt or two, which is the equivalent of no more than 2 to 3 ml or one-half teaspoon. Warm the oil and distribute it across both hands. With two hands placed on one foot at a time, you will begin to work the energy of the feet through as an entirety. Use circular and spiraling motions for your footwork. All movement is initiated with the center of the hands rather than the fingers. Think of cupping the foot between your two palms while sending spirals of light into the foot. Fingers, too, should be cupped rather than splayed out in a manner that directs your healing energy work away from the foot. As you work the feet with intention to relieve any tension, you also increase the possibility for freer flow of energy and, therefore, healing.

Although both the Provider and the Partner participate in a healing session, the Provider is the active electrode that draws forth energy of healing and the Partner is the passive electrode that receives the energy during the SEF treatment. The SEF Provider's intention is important in establishing these states by focusing on the Partner's needs while managing their own so that their needs do not become the focus either consciously or unconsciously.

Engage the mind as well as the heart and use your senses to observe very closely your Partner's energetic, physical, and emotional responses. This establishes a state of consciousness in the healing space created for manifesting the expression of your intention. During an SEF treatment, that intention centers on the healing work of the Partner. However, because the Provider is an electrode for channeling light and positive clear intention for healing as energy flow, the Provider also receives the benefit of the healing energy that flows through them as a result of delivering comfort and care to another. This is an ablution and anointing for the Provider that is in my experience just as, if not more, energizing than what one experiences as the recipient of SEF.

Let this teaching serve as a barometer for your development in SEF skills. One way that you can measure your development is whether you are energized and healed of your own concerns as a result of focusing on another's comfort and giving your offering with full awareness and pure heart. As you purify your heart—which is to be able to hold the love for another without the interference of your own needs, desires, beliefs and thoughts—you will experience the healing power of loving kindness in active service to others. SEF, with its specific techniques for moving energy flow, is one of the best healing art forms in which to learn some of these ancient healing principles.

Another one of the most important principles is that of keeping both hands on the feet. The two hands of the Provider are the conductor of the energy of love from the heart to the Partner. The use of the two hands in SEF delivers a *wholeness current* balancing the flow of energy (yin/yang; Alpha/Omega; plus/minus). This wholeness current is the channel for the signal that is sent to the brain and the blueprint. The use of two hands in a harmony of moving energy flow in the feet creates an opportunity for a release of fohat. Fohat is life-giving spiritual fire that can be released through actions and the spoken word, such as the invocation done before the ablution. It is the "bridge by which the ideas existing in the 'Divine Thought' are impressed on cosmic substance....Fohat is the dynamic energy of Cosmic Ideation...the guiding power of all manifestation...the mysterious link between mind and matter, the animating principle electrifying every atom into life."[16]

It was fun to watch fohat in action with Oma and Charles. I remember watching beads of perspiration form on Charles's forehead as he would work the feet strongly with his knuckles. His heart was fully activated when he gave a Foot Zone Therapy treatment. It was as if he was burning up the blockages with the powerful

---

16 (Blavatsky, 1888, p. II. 86)

energy that moved through his body. Then his heart, as the center for the light of healing, would leave his hands. From Oma, I learned the power of fohat in concentration on the feet. She would look so deeply at them, giving me permission and invitation to do the same. SEF is a chalice for the power of fohat that promises potential for the following to occur:

- Relaxation
- Increased adaptation response while decreasing stress response
- Restored energy flow and circulation, thereby increasing the natural ability of cells to excrete waste products of metabolic processes
- Assisting in the reestablishment of homeostasis, a tendency toward equilibrium rather than a fixed state
- Establishing a clearer connection with Earth through the electrode of the feet

APPROACH

What makes each SEF treatment and each Provider different is their approach or the way in which they express fohat, the way they move the energy in the feet, and the effort with which they do so. The fourth "A" of preparation for a basic SEF treatment is approach. Every healing art form has its tenets and designs that make it what it is. Your personal approach is your repertoire that you draw from to provide a healing service to another. The greater the repertoire or palette of approaches you possess, the better you are able to meet the needs of the diverse families and communities in which we live. This does not mean that more modalities are needed as much as a greater repertoire and palette within a single modality are needed. I learn something new about the approach to SEF from every client I treat. Every person's feet inform the next treatment and help to build my knowledge and understanding of best SEF practice.

At the center of the approach to best practice is *flow*. The SEF Provider's flow must communicate with the Partner's flow. There must be a harmony of exchange of energy to which the Provider adapts his/her hand movements to promote the flow of energy in the feet in general (as when working the feet through) or in specific fields or points representing the hologram of an organ. Because the focus is flow, we come to realize very quickly that an SEF treatment is more than pushing points on the feet. Anyone can "ring the bell" for an organ's energy field if they know some anatomy and hold an understanding of the hologram. But moving the energy in a way that complements physiology and energy patterns of the unique person is more challenging. This is the healing art that is SEF.

Just as Monet's paintings are more than his brush strokes, Thoreau's musings about Walden Pond more than the words on the page, and Ruth St. Denis's dances more than steps or movements, SEF is more than pushing points. SEF, like all art, is that which connects or integrates the elements manifesting in form. SEF is energy flow. As a professional dancer in the 1980s in New York, I learned from one of my favorite ballet master teachers, Finis Jhung, that *dance* is not a position or movement but what "happens between two movements." He was right; dance is flow. So I continue to work from this premise of seeking flow in my dance and all of my life work. I applied this wisdom teaching early on in foot reflexology and it has come to be an integral part of teaching and learning SEF. Oma always chastised her students that foot reflexology was not "pushing points." SEF's focus on energy flow establishes a beginning point for the development of an approach to the work that emphasizes the connections between points as the Provider's expression of Self in loving response to the need of the Partner. In an SEF treatment, as in dance, to set the matrix for flow to emerge, we begin with breath. Likewise, dance and movement begin with breath and then foot positions. After breath in SEF, we move to learning hand positions and holds.

Opening the Sinuses and the Breath

When we focus on breath, we focus on energy flow. It is that simple. When we get stuck in anything, from life to SEF, the first step is to breathe. We start life, in fact, with breath and the first one is really more of a gasp! Inhalation and exhalation are similar in movement to the tides in the sea. They come and go like a swooping bird rather than a crack of lightning. The ease with which we breathe impacts the flow of light and energy through the chakras or energy centers, and blood and qi through body organs and systems. One reason for this is the diaphragm muscle, the conductor of breathing that crosses all 10 zones of the body. This means that from the perspective of the hologram and energy flow, the diaphragm muscle affects the entirety.

When we become stressed, our breathing becomes shallower. The purpose of the breathing preparation is to help the Partner and yourself release tension in the body and facilitate centering. One of the major impediments to proper breathing is the health of the sinuses. Fortunately, the sinuses often open easily as a result of the footbath, anointing with eucalyptus oil, and ablution. But when you begin to work the feet of the person on the table, it is helpful to do preliminary work with the sinuses. The technique for this is called "milking." To milk the sinus areas, first locate the head area, which is found in the toes on the SEF chart. To milk the sinuses, you will use the thumb and first finger to milk the webbing between each toe. [*See Figure 1-4*]

With the first finger on the top of the foot and the thumb under the foot, gently engage and pull the energy from the middle of the metatarsal toward the center of the webbing between each of the toes. The full sinus

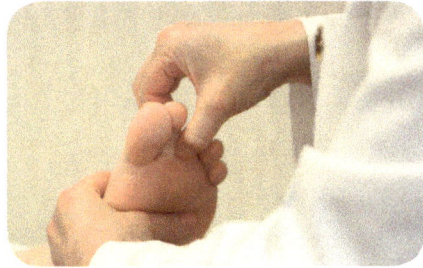

1-4   MILKING THE SINUSES

treatment is conducted during the basic treatment. This action serves to begin the opening. When working the sinus area, two hands are working on one foot to deliver the wholeness current. The other foot is covered with the towel.

A Repertoire of Holds, Positions, and Techniques

Hand positions and holds are expressions of your personal repertoire in SEF. As you grow in technique for identifying and "ringing the bells" of organ points (the focus of Chapter 2), so too should you focus on expanding your repertoire for knowing how, when, and where to hold the feet, and what hand positions to use to do so in a manner that ultimately supports the goals of the SEF treatment. The following are the holds and positions commonly used in SEF that will also be referred to in Chapter 2: *Initiating the Basic SEF Treatment.* Begin by standing or sitting at the end of the table facing the feet of your Partner. Your initial position is "place." Notice that your left hand is on their right foot and vice versa. This is important to realize when land marking the hologram and may take a little getting used to at first.

Calming Hold

The calming hold [*See Figure 1-5*] is used when the SEF Provider wants to send light into the feet or a specific point and to help the Partner transmute any discomfort that they may have experienced. Also consider a calming hold while listening to the Partner reveal important health pattern information. The hands are held in position and although they

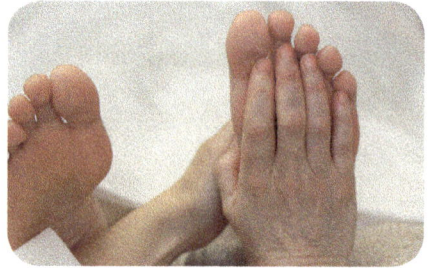

1-5 CALMING HOLD

may not move much, they are still very active energetically speaking.

There are a number of positions used when calming the feet or a point. The basic position is two hands on one foot with the right hand delivering energy to the sole of the foot (palm to sole) and the left hand behind the foot or point receiving or drawing the energy toward it. Another calming hold can be done with the palm of each hand connected with the energy center found in the top of the foot at the height of the instep. Gently pull the feet toward your heart to maintain a full connection with the feet. Hold until you feel muscle release and/or increase pulse or energy in the chakra or field.

Palm-to-Sole Hold

The palm-to-sole hold [*See Figure 1-6*] is a calming hold that engages the entirety and also specifically energizes the kidneys/adrenal glands, ears, and eyes. Sit at the feet and place one palm on each foot with

your fingertips tucked under slightly so that they engage the base of the Partner's toes (eyes/ears field). Your palm sits snugly over the sole of the foot with your thumb wrapped to the inside of the Partner's feet.

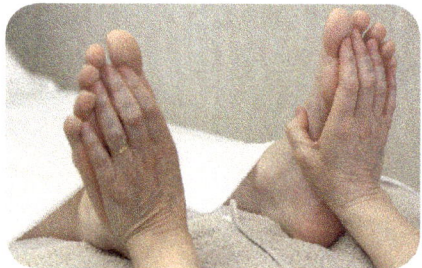

1-6 PALM-TO-SOLE HOLD

The tip of your thumb is then in position to sit gently on the kidney and adrenal field, which sits below the waistline to the inside of the spine. Hold until you feel muscle release and/or increase pulse or energy in the chakra or field.

Kidney-Charging Hold

To charge the kidneys, start in palm-to-sole hold. [*See Figure 1-7*] Take one hand off the foot and place your hand on the center back calf muscle of the leg, which you are still holding. Ideally keep your hands in position until you feel a pulse beating at the same rhythm in both the foot and calf. The "charging" action includes visualizing the drawing down of light from your higher Self, through the top of the head, then in to the heart and out through your hands into the foot and calf of your Partner. This hold is a chalice for a gift of light to our Partner's kidneys. The kidneys are the site for what is referred to in Traditional Chinese Medicine (TCM) as the natal jing (energy). Natal jing is like a bank account. Once the jing or money is spent, it is gone. More money or energy can be deposited, but it is not natal jing. In TCM, it is understood that people typically tap their jing stores as they age, hence increasing the likelihood of a health pattern called "yin deficiency." The jing account can also be spent through lifestyle choices such as stressful jobs, substance misuse, and excessive or promiscuous sexual activity. I discovered the power of this compassionate action hold for the kidneys when I was working with Oma in her clinic years ago. Oma agreed.

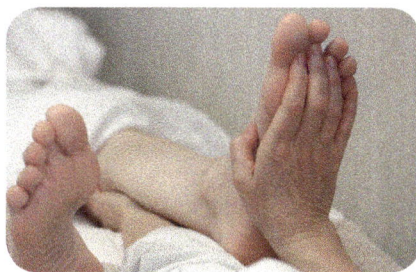

1-7 KIDNEY-CHARGING HOLD

Solar Plexus Hold

Another calming/compassion-ate action hold is the solar plexus hold. [*See Figure 1-8*] This hold is also used for the solar plexus treatment. The solar plexus is a nerve center in the core of the abdomen under the sternum.

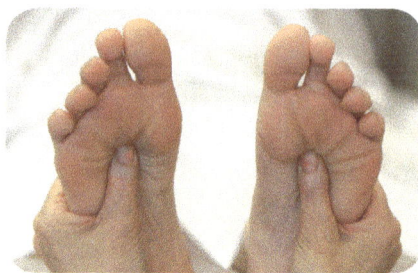

1-8 SOLAR PLEXUS HOLD

On the feet, it is a large field in the center of the foot under the ball of the foot. The solar plexus works in concert with the diaphragm muscle and is therefore sensitive to changes in breathing patterns.

To calm the solar plexus, place the flat distal tips of the thumb of each hand up and into the solar plexus point under the ball of the foot. Instruct the Partner to breathe and "let go" of or "release" any muscle tension they feel. I do not tell people to "relax" as my observation of the response is that the person always tenses the muscles more. Push in and instruct your Partner to breathe in for a count of eight. Then release the point slightly and instruct the Partner to lift the ribs and sustain the breath for eight counts; then release the thumb fully over the count of eight without taking the tip of the thumb off the solar plexus point; instruct the Partner to drop their jaw and allow the breath to release with a pop of the lips (like a balloon). Keep the thumb in place and instruct the Partner to push the breath out of the lungs fully for the final count of eight. Repeat the four-part breathing of eight counts each two to three times. Finish the hold with instruction to breathe in and out and then normally. If a client has asthma or other breathing concerns, you can do the four-part breathing with four counts instead of eight. This solar plexus hold is compassionate action because the SEF Provider can actually draw out the tension with the thumbs and release the energy into the violet fire and the Earth on behalf of the Partner.

Toe Rotation and Twist

Toe rotation and twisting are techniques used to release tension in the head and neck area and the ring muscles of the eyes. [*See Figure 1-9*] Rotate the great toe by stabilizing the base of the toe with one hand and

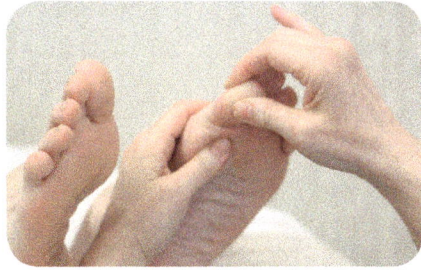

1-9   TOE ROTATION AND TWIST

holding the top of the great toe with the other hand. You may need to use the towel so that your hands do not slip when rotating the toe. The motion should simulate that which happens when we gently lift our head away from the spine and rotate our head and neck. Lift the toe first away from the foot and then circle the toe one way and then another. This rotation can be completed with all toes. It is followed with a gentle twisting action. Twist an individual toe by holding it with the thumb on one side and the other fingers behind. Squeeze to maintain contact with the energy in each toe. Twist each toe, working your way to the tip of the toe. This action affects the head and sinus areas and is specifically helpful in releasing tension in the ring muscles of the eyes.

Thumb Walking

Thumb walking is a technique of major importance for the SEF treatment. [*See Figure 1-10*] It is used primarily to move energy along the spine. The nervous system and all of the body organs are impacted by the flow of energy through the spine. Spine walking sends a series of signals

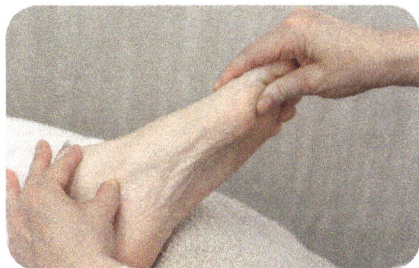

1-10   THUMB WALKING

and delivers a wholeness current from the base of the spine to the head. Before positioning your hands on the feet to practice thumb walking, do this experiment. Sit at a table and stretch your arms in front of you with your hands flat on the table. [*See Figure 1-11*]

Look at the position of your thumbs closely. This is the proper thumb position for spine walking. Notice that the outside edge and upper outer corner of the thumb are in contact with the table. The inside of the thumb is not. It is facing you. While still on the table, bend your thumb at the first joint and then straighten it. This action causes your thumb to move forward (away from your body) in small stitches like a sewing machine. Each time that you bend your thumb, you take a small stitch or "bite." When you release, your thumb will naturally walk forward. Now as you practice the bend-and-straighten action, add another important action. When you practice thumb walking on the spine, from #11 to #14, bend at the knuckle to "ring the bell" for each vertebra along the spine. This means that you will go in toward the spine points with the outer tip of your thumb, and then release and repeat. Each signal, as a release of fohat and light, is released up the spine. The location of the parts of the spine and walking the spine will be detailed further in Chapter 2.

Energetically, each time you send a signal to the spine or any organ through thumb walking or the other techniques, you are sending an action of the power, wisdom, and love of the heart. The action associated with contacting a field in the hologram and sending a signal for that body organ or system expresses the power of

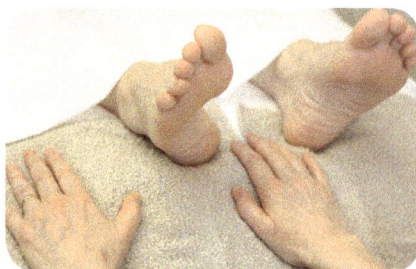

1-11 PROPER THUMB POSITION

the heart. The color associated with power is blue. In an SEF treatment, visualize blue when sending a signal. The color associated with the love of the heart expressed in sending a signal is rose pink. When sending a signal, visualize the hand that is holding the foot as bathed in pink light. When we combine pink and blue as we do in sending a signal, we have an overall action of the color violet. Violet is the color of transmutation and freedom. This is why we hypothesize that the SEF treatment is a transformative treatment. It operationalizes the violet fire in a very accessible healing action.

At first, many people who learn SEF contort their hands to work the spine. However, if you place your hands on your Partner's feet as you did on the table, you will find the thumb-walking technique to be much easier to do. If you feel tied up in knots during thumb walking, you probably are and may be sending knotty energy to your Partner. Stop and adjust your stance. Start in "place." Move both hands to one foot. The inside hand is your left hand when working on your Partner's left foot and your right hand when working on their right foot. To walk the spine, you will use your inside hand and support the foot with your outside hand. Practice thumb walking on your steering wheel while sitting at a stoplight. Or practice on your own hand. Concentrate on making smaller stitches or bites and sending a signal only with the thumb while the other fingers are supporting, not pushing a point unknowingly. While practice begins on the spine, the thumb walking technique is used on energy fields for other organs such as the large intestine located in the soles of the feet.

Spine Stretch

After walking the spine, perform a spine stretch. [*See Figure 1-12*] Clasp your fingers together around a single foot with the interlaced area of the fingers over the spine. Hold and stretch the spine as you

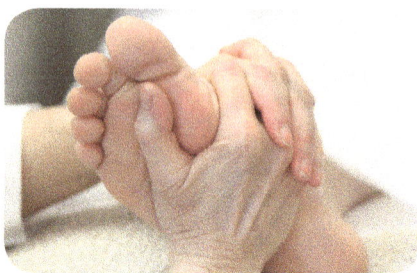

1-12 SPINE STRETCH

gently pull the foot toward your heart with shoulders down. Maintain proper posture during the SEF treatment, particularly during techniques when you support the weight of the Partner's leg.

Egyptian / Cradle Hold and Position

The Egyptian hold refers to the treatment position observed in the glyph found in the Egyptian tomb referred to in the Introduction. [*See Figure 1-13*] For this hold and position, the SEF Provider walks to the side of the Partner's feet, and faces away from the head of the Partner. The Provider's hands deliver signals now by wrapping around from the side or back to the sole of the foot. Holding the foot in Egyptian position to your heart is a wonderful Egyptian calming hold. Your arms are in natural position to support the weight of the foot and leg and allow the whole leg to release tension. I also refer to this hold as the "cradle hold."

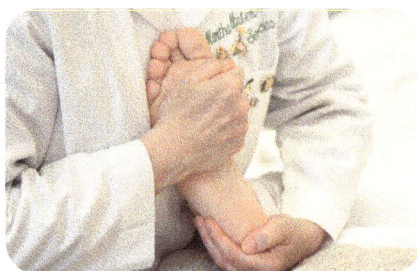

1-13 EGYPTIAN / CRADLE HOLD

60

Hook and Back-Up Position and Technique

Hook and back-up is a technique used for sending a signal
from either the original place
or the Egyptian positions. [*See
Figure 1-14*] Hook and back-up
is used for certain hard-to-
reach points on the great toe,

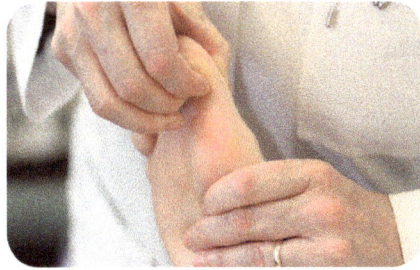

1-14   HOOK AND BACK-UP POSITION

for example. After sending the signal with the thumb (place position)
or second or third finger tip (Egyptian), lift the point up and back
while maintaining pressure.

Heart Hold

Place the right palm over the heart area (the ball of the foot) on one foot
and the left palm behind the foot. [*See Figure 1-15 A and B*] Visualize
and hold until you feel muscle release or increase in energy flow. The
heart hold can also be done with one hand on each foot. As you face
the Partner, place the palm of your left hand over the heart area on
the Partner's right foot and your right palm over the heart area on the
Partner's left foot.

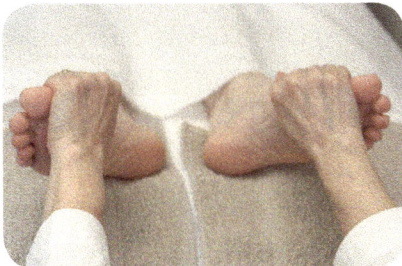

1-15A   HEART HOLD

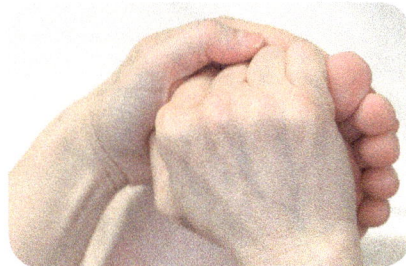

1-15B   HEART HOLD

Finger Wave

The tissue on the top of the feet is considerably thinner than on the soles of the feet. Thumb walking along certain points is helpful, but many of the organs, such as the lymphatic system and the breast, are

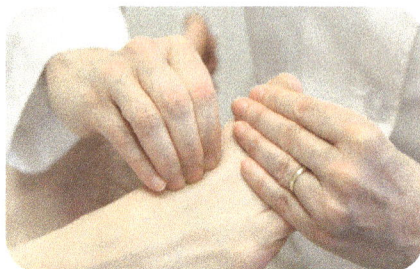
1-16   FINGER WAVE

represented in larger areas on the top of the feet. Sending a signal in these areas can be accomplished with the finger wave. [*See Figure 1-16*] Place the middle three fingertips together and perform the same walking motion as is done in spine walking. The finger wave can be used when it is not necessary to go as deeply into the tissues of the foot and a more superficial action suffices.

Spirals

Spirals and circles are really important actions in SEF. [*See Figure 1-17*] They are the equivalent of a massage-like action, which Oma always referred to as "dessert!" Just as dessert is served after a meal,

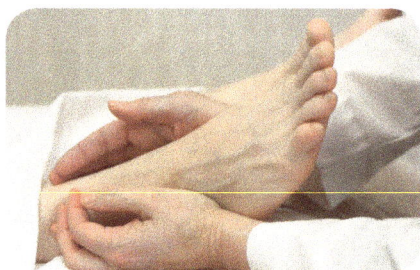
1-17   SPIRALS

spirals are typically done after sending a signal. Sending a signal can be intense and even painful. The spiral action on the foot after that release of energy can help to dissipate the pain and associated tension activated with the signal response. Any part of the foot and ankle can benefit from spirals. Two hands are always used to make spirals. To do an ankle spiral, hold the heel with one hand and circle the whole foot with the other hand. Another ankle spiral technique is cupping the ankle on each side with the palm of each hand and rotating the palms while moving them around the ankle joint. As the foot relaxes, it will respond more freely to the rotation.

Spirals are three-dimensional movement whereas other motions in massage are two-dimensional (horizontal and vertical). The third dimension that spirals bring to the SEF treatments is sagittal or forward-back motion. Each spiral action sends a signal that can move the Partner forward. Now we are ready to move forward into the next phase—*Initiating the Basic SEF Treatment.*

Alexandersson, O. (1997). *Living Water: Viktor Schauberger and the Secrets of Natural Energy.* Bath, UK: Gateway Books.

Becker, R., & Selden, G. (1998). *The Body Electric.* New York: William Morrow Paperbacks.

Bible - King James Version. (1972). United States: Thomas Nelson, Publishers.

Blavatsky, H. (1888). *The Secret Doctrine: The Synthesis of Science, Religion, and Philosophy.* London: The Theosophical Publishing Co.

Csikszentmihalyi, M. (1990). *Flow: The Psychology of Optimal Experience.* New York: Harper Perennial.

Diamandopoulos, A., Vlachos, J., & Marketos, S. (1997). "The Survival of the Ritualistic Over the 'Scientific' Element of Hydrotherapy in Greece." *History of Psychiatry*, 8(29 pt 1), 21-35.

Diamond, J. (1979). *Behavioral Kinesiology: How to Activate Your Thymus and Increase Your Life Energy.* New York: Harper & Row.

Knox, W. (1950). John 13.1-30. *Harvard Theological Review*, 43(2), 161-163.

Liao, W., Landis, C., Lentz, M., & Chiu, M.-J. (2005). "Effects of Foot Bathing on Distal-Proximal Skin Temperature Gradient in Elders." *International Journal of Nursing Studies*, 42(7), 717-722.

Libster, M., & McNeil, B. A. (2009). *Enlightened Charity: The Holistic Nursing Care, Education and Advices Concerning the Sick of Sister Matilda Coskery, (1799-1870).* http://www.GoldenAppleHealingArts.com: Golden Apple Publications.

Sung, E.-J., & Tochihara, Y. (2000). "Effects of Bathing and Hot Footbath on Sleep in Winter." *Journal of Physiological Anthropology and Applied Human Science*, 19(1), 21-27.

Weiss, H. (1979). "Foot Washing in the Johannine Community." *Novum Testamentum*, 21(4), 298-325.

CHAPTER TWO

Initiating the Basic SEF Treatment

Given the length of the last chapter on preparation for a basic SEF treatment, you might now be wondering how long a treatment actually takes! Learning SEF or any healing modality from a two-dimensional book does make the process appear longer than it actually is. But in reality, much of the energetic preparation described in Chapter 1 takes place at the speed of light! Once you develop the momentum or habits of the 4 A's of attunement, ablution, anointing, and approach, you will find that the preparation for a basic treatment that includes a five-minute footbath takes about 15 minutes.

After disengaging from the effect of daily effluvia, beginning your attunement, and dawning your protection through anointing, you and your Partner are prepared to connect with the divine blueprint of wholeness. While all that has been done to this point has begun the process of activating energy flow, the purpose of the next phase—initiating the basic SEF treatment—is moving energy: organ system by organ system. The SEF treatment addressed in this chapter and Chapter 3 is "basic" not because it is easy or mundane, but because it is a starting point. The system-by-system treatment described here represents the foundational knowledge that you must have to do SEF. It is the platform from which your own creativity and inner wisdom can build your "unique techniques" for engaging energy flow in the hologram of the feet.

Just as life begins with a heartbeat, the process of engaging the blueprint for each organ system begins with the heart. You enter into the energetic center of the blueprint through the hidden chamber of the heart. This entering into the inner self is a process and a practice similar to prayer, meditation, reflection, centering, and contemplation. The only difference is that in SEF the entering is done with a Partner. Jesus the Christ, who was a great healer, taught the action of the hidden chamber, "When thou prayest, enter into thy closet, and when thou hast shut thy door, pray to the Father which is in secret; and thy Father which seeth in secret shall reward thee openly."[1] He then went on to teach forgiveness as invoked through recitation of the Lord's Prayer followed by a teaching on "treasures in heaven." In SEF, the treasures in heaven can be likened to the divine blueprint that we access for wholeness and healing. Jesus said:

> Lay not up for yourselves treasures upon earth, where moth and rust doth corrupt, and where thieves break through and steal; But lay up for yourselves treasures in heaven, where neither moth nor rust corrupt, and where thieves do not break through nor steal: For where your treasure is, there will your heart be also. The light of the body is the eye: if therefore thine eye be single, thy whole body shall be full of light.[2]

This teaching is important in that it affirms what teachers of the healing arts know to this day. No one—physician, nurse, family member, or therapist—has the power to penetrate or "corrupt" that

---

1   (Bible, 1972, Matt 6:6)
2   (Bible, 1972, Matt 6: 19-22)

which is stored at the level of the divine. The blueprint is incorruptible and is accessed through one's connection with the "heaven" world. This connection is possible through the light of the eye and the treasure of the heart.

The heart, called Chitta, which is the "seat of bliss"—or ananda in yogic teachings[3]—is a central receiving point of connection with our treasures in heaven, the blueprint. The "action of Attraction, as the Omnipotent love in the core of the heart"[4] is the central focus for the descent of the light of God, the Creator of the blueprint. This descent of light, first into the center of the heart—the hidden chamber—is what is visualized in an SEF treatment. This supports the infusion of the body and its organs "on earth" in the material plane with love and light, the magnet of attraction for wholeness—as above, so below.

The basic SEF treatment uses physical touching of the feet and its associated hologram of the entirety to access this spiritual connection with the receptive heart as one of the seven major energy centers in the body. These major energy centers are referred to in Sanskrit as *patalas* or chakras. Biblically, the seven major chakras are referred to as the "seven golden candlesticks" that are the "seven churches."[5] Sri Yukteswar, an Indian saint, yogi, and scholar, identified these seven shining places in the body as manifesting in the brain and spine; more specifically: the brain, medulla oblongata, cervical spine, dorsal spine, lumbar spine, sacrum, and coccyx.[6] While SEF is in full agreement with this teaching of the focuses of light in the body along the central nervous system (brain and spine), its chakras are identified with major

---

3   (Yukteswar, 1990 (Originally published 1949), p. 35)
4   (Yukteswar, 1990 (Originally published 1949), p. 36)
5   (Bible, 1972, Rev 1:12,13,16,20)
6   (Yukteswar, 1990 (Originally published 1949), p. 91)

endocrine glands, which are innervated within the zones related to the seven candlesticks of the ancient wisdom teaching. Endocrine glands secrete hormones, which are catalysts for changes in the body that regulate all functions and physical and mental constructive powers.

THE CHAKRA CONNECTION BETWEEN ENDOCRINE AND ENERGY SYSTEMS

As light energy is received into the body, it enters first through the nervous system and the chakras associated with it. The chakras are like cups that are positioned upright toward the sun so that when the light rays descend into the energy field of the person, they can be held. Light descends first into the heart and then the pulse of life force is distributed from the heart to the other major chakras and then out to the rest of the body. In SEF, working the chakras is done through the energy field of the major endocrine glands associated with those energy centers.

In the 1980s, I found Oma's teaching on working the energy centers through the feet quite natural. I am not sure why this was so. Perhaps it was my understanding of the physiology of the body and the flow of energy from my training and experience as a dancer that never made me question the connection she made with the feet. As I have worked over the years with the teaching and worked the feet in the way I am about to share with you, I have found it to be one of the most, if not *the* most, profound teachings in the healing arts around the globe. I have come to realize what a privilege and gift it was to have been given the opportunity to have learned this at such an early age. In honor of that privilege, I state as a nurse-scientist with full confidence that while we may not fully comprehend the workings of this treatment with our outer minds, I am completely humbled by its positive effects on health and healing. In this first part of the basic treatment, SEF meets chakra science and tradition through the heart, head, and hands. We have spoken of the heart. This is now the teaching that will engage your head and hands as the instruments for making the chakra connection.

THE SEVEN CANDLESTICKS

One of the most preeminent teachers on the ancient wisdom in Hindu/Yoga tradition is Paramahansa Yogananda. He was sent by Sri Yukteswar to bring knowledge of the "royal science of God-realization" to the West. In his publication translating and teaching *The Bhagavad Gita*, he quotes the book of Genesis in the Bible:

> And 'God said, Let there be light: and there was light.' That is God's thought vibrated into the light of cosmic life or cosmic prana; and cosmic prana was further materialized into electrons, protons, atoms, molecules, cells and matter. The cosmic thought of God thus first materialized as the cosmic prana or life force of light, and finally as all matter of the macrocosm. The body of man is a microcosm of the Lord's creation. The microcosmic human body is a composite of the individual's soul and life force.[7]

This is the spiritual essence of the application or manifestation of the teaching of bringing the blueprint of wholeness into manifestation and why a very suitable invocation for an SEF treatment is, "Let there be light!" It is light that nourishes body, mind, and spirit, and it is the ability to hold that light drawn into our bodies from our source that is a function of the health of the chakras and their related glands.

---

7   (Yogananda, 1995, p. 570)

A "healthy" chakra is one that is free from effluvia. For example, in the case of the heart chakra, effluvia or impurities might manifest as or be due to hatred. It is hard to know which comes first. Does an impurity such as hatred cause the effluvia to collect around the heart chakra or does the imbalance in the heart chakra (perhaps due to karmic circumstance) create the magnet for the effluvia? The patterns observed from helping so many people over time suggest that both can and do occur. An important teaching people find very helpful is that these impurities that gather around the chakras are not always due to personal circumstance and choice. They are also the result of energies taken on from others as well as from the planet. For example, someone may take on or share the hatred energy of their spouse or ethnic group. In either case, personal or planetary, effluvia around the chakras can be transmuted and changed into light. What appears as dark soot around the chakra can be scrubbed away through a number of practices. Two such practices are visualization and invocation.

In the first part of the basic SEF treatment, the chakras are accessed through the hologram in the feet by sending a signal from the energy fields of the related endocrine gland and the spine. We work the energy field of the gland while visualizing the chakra in its pure state—that is what it is at the level of the blueprint. The blueprint sits in the etheric plane of consciousness; this is the plane of the pure light as opposed to the astral realm, which is influenced, if not tainted, by human desires and passions. Working at the level of the etheric blueprint affords an element of spiritual protection to the SEF Provider and Partner alike whereby the purifying effect of the ablution of the energy field is better sustained and the vortex or opening that is created is not filled with discordant thought forms. It is customary practice in SEF to draw forth from the pure spring of the higher Self with which we connect through the power of the seven chakras.

Seven is an important number to work with in the healing arts. It holds great significance in religions, cosmologies, and in many cultural traditions, such as are found written in the *Pistis Sophia* of the Gnostics, the *Kabala* of the Jews, and the *Vedas* of the Hindus. An excellent summary of the history of seven in those teachings can be found in *The Secret Doctrine*[8] by Helena Blavatsky, who founded the Theosophical Society in the late nineteenth century with the Mahatmas Morya and Kuthumi. She writes:

> *Thus Number Seven, as a compound of 3 and 4, is the factor element in every religion, because it is the factor element in nature ... Saptaparna. Such is the name given in Occult phraseology to man. It means ...a seven-leaved plant ... The T or T (tau), formed from the figure 7, and the Greek letter Γ (gamma), was ("cross and circle") the symbol of life and of life eternal: of earthly life, because r (gamma) is the symbol of the Earth (gaia) : and of 'life eternal,' because the figure 7 is the symbol of the same life linked with the divine life ...a triangle and a quaternary, the symbol of septenary man.*[9]

Connecting the seven major chakras with their associated glands occurs within the overarching platform for light, life, and unity represented in the number 7, the triangle (3) above, plus the square (4) below. The upper three chakras (the triangle) represent the treasures of spirit and that which is unchanging. The lower four represent matter, or that which changes. The heart chakra occupies the place of the nexus between that which is above—the throat, third eye, and crown chakras—and that which is below—the solar plexus, Seat-of-the-Soul, and Base-of-the-Spine chakras. Meditation upon these seven

---

8   (Blavatsky, 1888, pp. 598-641)
9   (Blavatsky, 1888, pp. 590 - 591)

chakras is a reflection on the ancient maxim, "As Above, So Below." The meditation on the seven chakras in SEF becomes a vehicle for the expression of the ancient wisdom and the drawing forth of the light of God in manifestation in man. The feet become the anchor for this work. Oma always speculated that Jesus would have known these ancient wisdom teachings and therefore knew that when he washed the disciples' feet, he was also "aligning" their chakras to receive the descent of light—"As Above, So Below." Light from God is one, infinite energy, all one.

THE TAU SPIRAL

Begin the SEF meditation on the tau with anchoring the light in the heart. The heart then distributes that light in a pattern of an expanding spiral to the other six chakras. *[See Figure 2-1]* The working of the feet follows this same pattern; therefore, begin at the heart, then move to the closest of the upper triad—the throat chakra; then spiral to the first chakra below the heart, which is the solar plexus chakra. From the solar plexus chakra, draw the energy up to the next chakra of the triad—the third eye—and then down to the Seat-of-the-Soul chakra. Move to the final chakra in the triad—the crown chakra—and then back down to the base-of- the-spine chakra, which is the final lower chakra. After working the base, you will walk up the spine drawing the light up the spine with you to anchor in the head at the third eye. In ancient healing traditions, it is taught that light within the energy field flows naturally up the spine to the crown and then anchors at the brow—the third eye.

When I worked with Oma, we tried a variety of patterns for working the chakras. For many years I worked a chakra on one foot and then on the other, most often starting at the base of the spine and

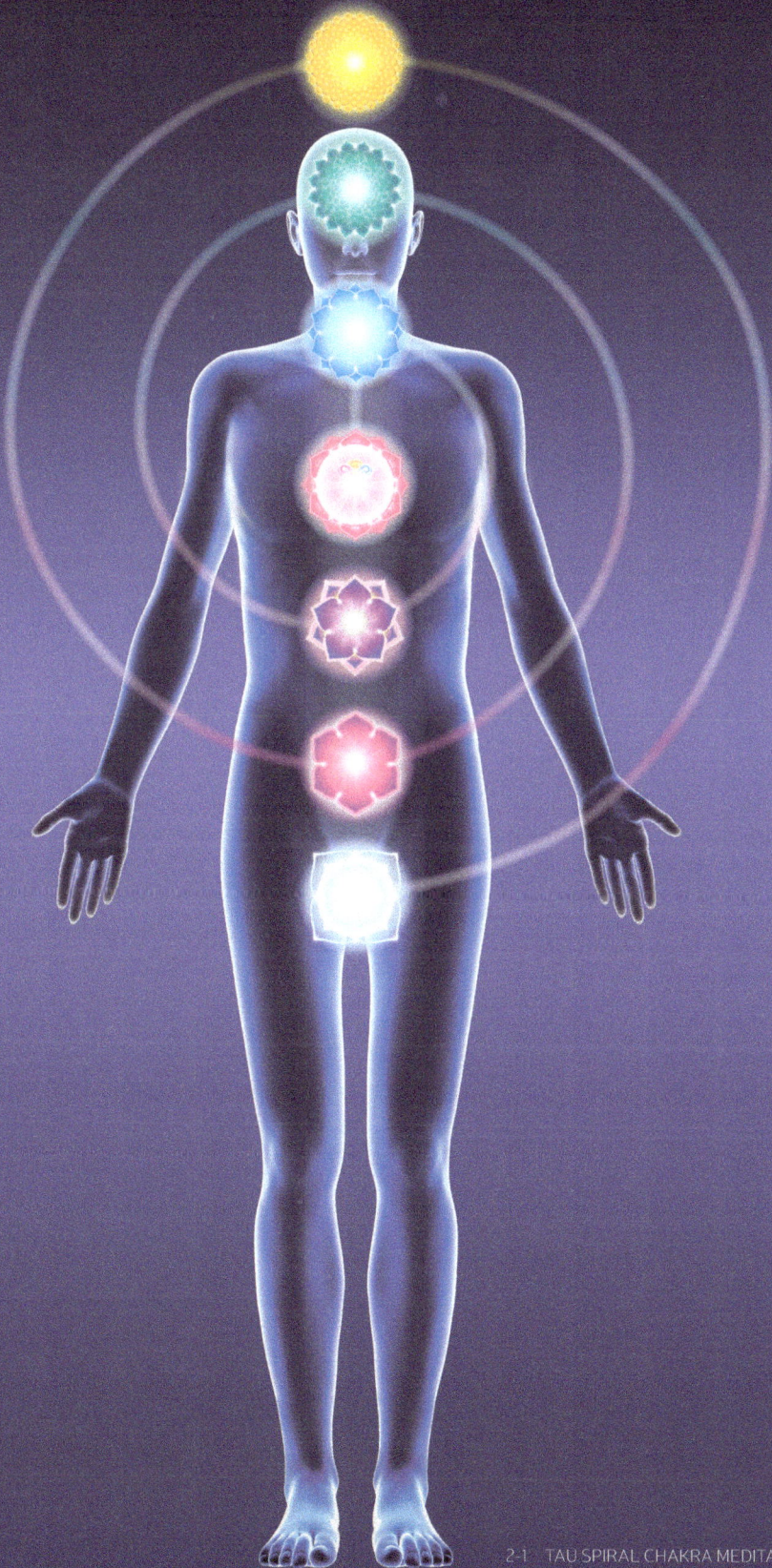

2-1 TAU SPIRAL CHAKRA MEDITATION

then working up to the crown. But the vision and inspiration for this Tau Spiral practice pattern described here, which I was inspired with some time ago, has never left me. It has only become more developed over time with the growth of understanding about the elements of creation and the power of the seven. The SEF Tau Spiral chakra meditation is done first on one foot and then on the other so that a complete spiral is created for each foot.

To send the signals for the chakras, you must locate the endocrine glands associated with each chakra. [*See Figure 2-2*] The chakra-gland connection is as follows:

Heart - Thymus gland behind the sternum at the center of the chest.

Throat - Thyroid gland located at the front lower part of the neck.

Solar Plexus - Adrenal gland located on the top of the kidney on the inside of the foot.

Third Eye - Pineal gland in the brain.

Seat-of-the-Soul - Pancreas located near the waistline marking on both feet.

Crown - Pituitary gland in the brain.

Base-of-the-Spine - Gonads (male) / uterus and ovaries (female).

Each of the chakras vibrates at a particular frequency, making each appear a particular color. There is a summary chart of the chakras at the end of this chapter. You will find on the following pages a description of each chakra, an artistic interpretation of how each appears in its pure state, and a description of the physiology of the related gland. Just as all chakras work in harmony, so too do the glands. When you touch one gland, you affect them all. In SEF, we focus on the seven

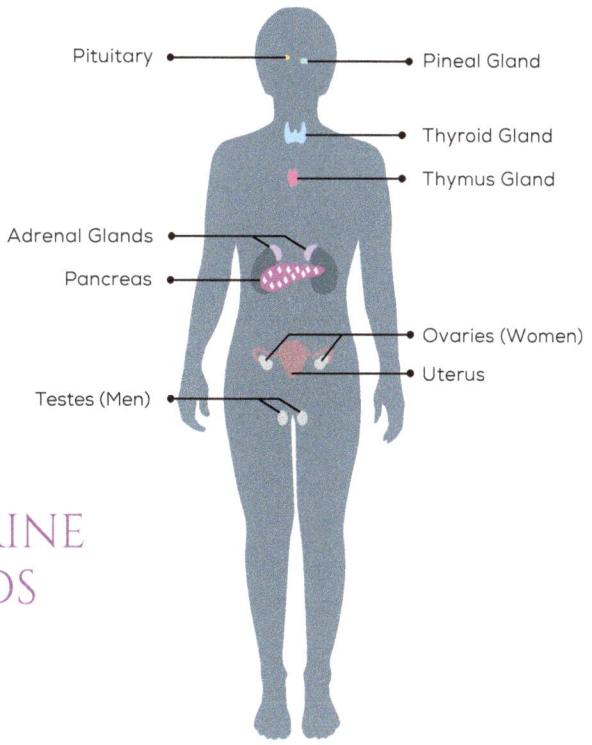

Pituitary

Pineal Gland

Thyroid Gland

Thymus Gland

Adrenal Glands

Pancreas

Ovaries (Women)

Uterus

Testes (Men)

ENDOCRINE GLANDS

Figure 2-2

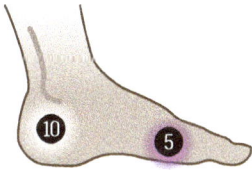

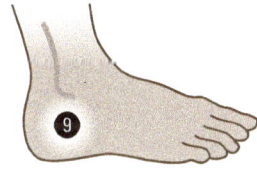

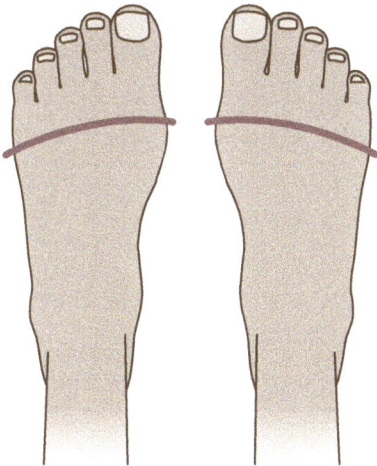

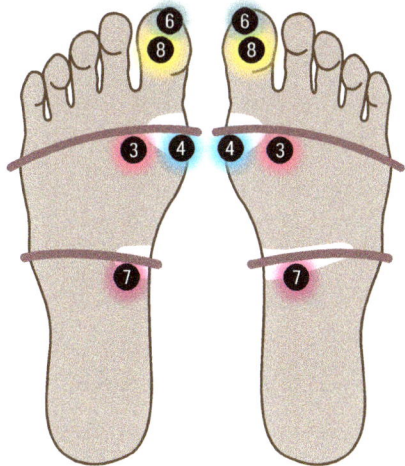

major chakras and glands, realizing that all energy centers that reside within the zones related to those seven will be affected as well. While in study we look at each individually in somewhat linear fashion, please remember that at their essence or white-fire core, the chakras are all one in the entirety. This is why at the center of each chakra, you will see in the pictures the inclusion of the white-fire core.

For the visualization of each chakra, begin by locating the associated gland in the feet. As you send the signal ("ring the bell") for that energy field, visualize the chakra as depicted here—spinning! In your mind's eye, visualize the spinning until you "see" the white-fire core at the center of the chakra. Those of you who do not have the developed inner sight can use the artwork for visualization. Hold only as long as it takes to construct the visualization. When the image of the white-fire core spinning has been constructed, release the point and move to the next chakra, following the spiral pattern as described above. This spinning action of the white- fire core throws off the sooty effluvia impinged on the chakra. This action prepares the chakra to hold the light descending from the person's higher Self. Visualize the violet fire around the chakra and gland, as was done during the ablution, and around your Partner's body and your own to transmute any potential or actual negative effects from the dislodged effluvia.

The SEF Provider serves as a catalyst for the process, but does not determine the flow of energy or light or transmutation. I liken the process to growing plants in a garden. We can do our best to get rid of the weeds and even water and fertilize the plant, but the growth of the plant is ultimately in God's hands. The growth of the human plant is the same. Ring the bell, visualize, bathe the person in violet fire and compassion, and then step back energetically. Allow nature to take its course and realize that all healing is manifest through the heart of the person. The quotient of light released for their use is determined within their relationship with their God/Creator. Over time you will find that your Partners are better able to hold more light in their chakras as manifest in the stories they relay about their health and energy levels. You can observe how they manifest greater and greater ability to maintain their health as well as any positive results from the SEF treatment.

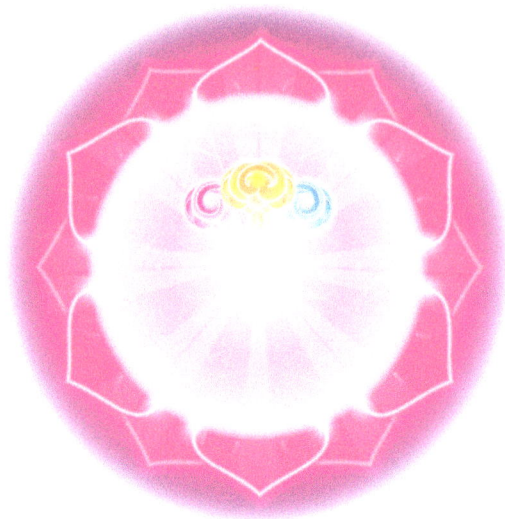

HEART

CHAKRA

The vibration of the heart chakra is love. At the center of the heart chakra is a threefold flame of pink, gold, and blue representing the divine virtues of love, wisdom, and power respectively. It is from the center of the heart and the threefold flame that concentric rings of energy, as depicted in paintings, labyrinths, and other aesthetic designs, are emitted. The action of purifying the heart also includes seeking greater balance and harmony in the heart as the manifestation of love, wisdom, and power. Love without wisdom and power is misplaced or selfish. Wisdom without love or power is unkind and mindless. Power without love and wisdom is cruel and reckless. The anchoring of these three divine virtues in the four lower planes of being is demonstrated in the vibration of 12 petals.

The heart chakra is associated with the thymus gland. The word thymus is derived from the Greek *thymos*, which denotes soul or feeling.

It is also thought that *thymos* once referred to breath. The thymus gland is located behind the sternum or breastbone. It is relatively large in the infant and decreases as we age. Although less is known about the gland than perhaps other glands, it is known that the thymus is related to the inhibition of the activity of the testicles and ovaries in children. "Castration causes persistent growth of the thymus. Removal of the thymus or its inhibition by X-ray hastens the development of the gonads."[10] The thymus hormones thymosin, thymopoietin, and serum thymic factor regulate several immune functions. Before and after birth, the thymus processes T-lymphocytes, the white blood cells involved in all of our body's cellular immunity. Environmental pollutants, radiation, and excessive debilitating stress (as opposed to creative tension) can weaken and diminish thymus function. Dr. John Diamond has worked for decades in his holistic psychotherapy and rehabilitation medicine practice exploring what restores and strengthens the thymus gland. He states that his work in Behavioral Kinesiology has shown that the thymus gland "monitors and regulates energy flow in the body."[11] In traditional Chinese medicine science, it is understood that the organ that regulates the flow of energy or qi in the body is the liver. However, from an SEF holographic perspective, I also agree with Dr. Diamond that energetically the heart chakra/thymus, as the recipient for the descent of light and qi, is therefore the regulator for it. His work includes testing the activation of the thymus gland to increase life energy through thumping or tapping the sternum, smiling, music, art, and lifestyle choices. Thump the thymus in the hologram of the feet; but, while doing so, instruct your Partner to tap their sternum too!

---

10   (Kapp, 1958, p. 39)
11   (Diamond, 1979, p. 28)

Note: As we begin to move into locating different organs and body systems in the hologram of the feet, it is recommended that you have the strongest knowledge of human anatomy as possible. I recommend that all SEF Providers complete a college-level anatomy and physiology course and own an excellent anatomy book. *The Anatomy Coloring Book*[12] is excellent because the action of coloring the beautiful drawings of the parts of the body establishes a deeper connection with the energetic patterns of the organs and systems in the body rather than rote memorization of body parts on a page.

---

12   (Kapit & Elson, 2001)

LOCATE AND WORK THE THYMUS GLAND

The thymus gland is #3 on the SEF Chart. It is located below the shoulder line and on the line between the first and second zones of both feet. Supporting the foot with your outer or inner hand, use your thumb-walking technique to feel for the point of maximum intensity in the energy field. You will feel a change in energy flow from the surrounding tissue. You may perceive this change in what you feel with your thumb as heat, warmth, a spark, or an energy surge. Roll your wrist forward so that the outer tip of your thumb rings the bell by connecting with the point of energy. You are pushing the point as you feel for the contact between your thumb tip and the strongest point of the energy field. The action is of power, wisdom, and love rather than mindless brute force without knowledge of the anatomy or physiology of the gland. This instruction applies to working the energy field of every organ. Visualize the pink color and 12 petals of the heart chakra spinning, the white-fire core spinning, and the violet fire consuming any effluvia. You might also choose to visualize a healthy thymus gland or white blood cells using pictures from an anatomy and physiology book.

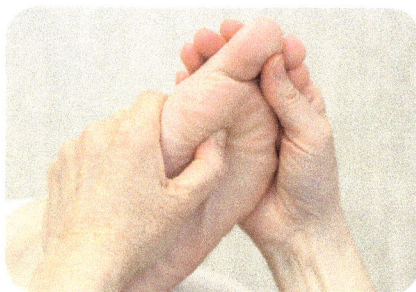

2-3 THYMUS/HEART CHAKRA

THROAT

CHAKRA

The vibration of the throat chakra is power. The color is blue, the color of a robin's egg. The chakra has 16 petals. Through the power center in the throat, we speak spirit or light into manifestation on the physical plane. If a person uses the name of God "I AM" and says, "I am _____" (fill in the blank), he/she is making that very statement true in his or her life. Much of the effluvia around the throat chakra is present as a result of the negative energy people put on themselves in the form of spoken limitations as to the power of the creator within. "I cannot do that. I AM too _____." Changing the way one speaks changes the momentum or habit of self-deprecation and limiting the power of God in one's life to manifest the blueprint.

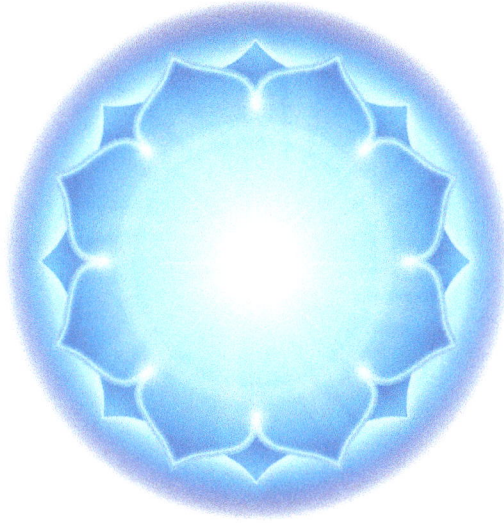

The throat chakra is related to the thyroid gland. While working the thyroid, have your Partner repeat a powerful mantra of protection and healing beginning with the statement, "I AM _____,"

which means "God within me is _____ ." Help your Partner re-pattern any negative momentums by accessing the power of the throat chakra.

The thyroid gland is a butterfly-shaped gland located at the base of the neck below the larynx or voice box. An energy-producing organ, it secretes thyroxin, which is an iodine-containing hormone that affects an increase in metabolism and energy production in the body. The gland regulates the level of iodine in the blood to be congruent with that of the sea. The liver is the greatest user of iodine in the body. The thyroid acts on the growth of skin (arsenic), hair, glands, and mucous membranes. It builds nerve and brain tissue (phosphorous) and secretes calcitonin, a blood calcium-lowering hormone. The thyroid is also active in the development of higher consciousness and psychic energy.

LOCATE AND WORK THE THYROID GLAND

The thyroid is #4 on the SEF Chart. It is located on both feet in zone 1 above the Cervical 7 landmark. Stabilize the foot with the outside hand and work the thyroid using the thumb-walking technique. Start inside the C7 field and walk horizontally across the thyroid field in zone 1 toward the beginning of zone 2. It usually takes about three to four bites (bend at knuckle and straighten) in adults, two in children, and one in infants. Visualize the blue color and 16 petals of the throat chakra spinning, the white-fire core spinning, and the violet fire consuming any effluvia. You might also choose to visualize a healthy thyroid gland using pictures from an anatomy and physiology book.

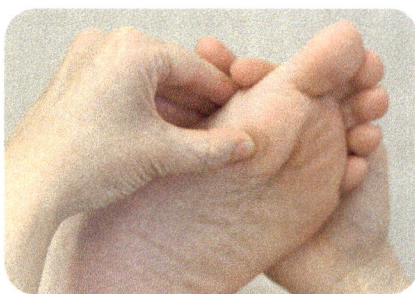

2-4 THYROID/THROAT CHAKRA

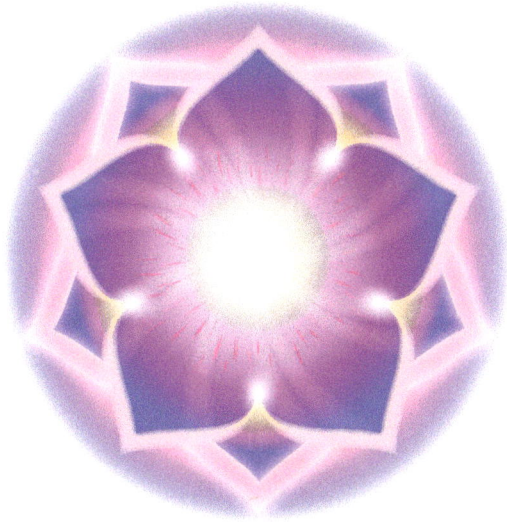

SOLAR PLEXUS

CHAKRA

The solar plexus chakra is a different energy field from the solar plexus nerve center in the center of the foot that was worked during the breathing exercise of the preparation phase. The vibration of the solar plexus chakra is peace. The color is purple and gold with ruby flecks. The chakra has 10 petals. Through the peace center, we engage emotion as "energy-in-motion," but realize the power of peace when the solar plexus can be stilled in the face of crisis and strong positive or negative emotions. The solar plexus and throat chakras are connected within the spiral. Jesus demonstrated this connection between chakras when he exhibited mastery of the solar plexus by making the invocation with his throat chakra, "Peace be still!" The ruby flecks represent the fire of the heart's desire necessary to calmly command the elements and maintain peace.

The solar plexus chakra is associated with the two adrenal glands that sit one upon each kidney. The kidney is in zone 2-3 on either side of the spine but the tricky part is to locate it and the adrenal glands on the hologram of the feet. Many charts, if not all charts I have seen, represent the kidneys on the bottom of the foot in zone 2-3, but this is not exactly correct. Charles Ersdal placed the kidney and adrenal glands just on the inner side of the foot next to the spine. He said that if the signal for the kidney was on the bottom of the foot, we would be urinating all day long. He had a point. However, if you look at what else is located in zone 2-3 at the waistline, you will understand that there are many organs that exist in the center of the body but that we feel our kidneys from the back near the spine and under the ribs. Therefore, I changed my practice in the 1990s after training with Charles because I shared his three-dimensional view for kidney and adrenal placement. Since then I have confirmed that while the other placement is not necessarily wrong, *it is easier to send a signal to the kidney and adrenal glands from the position near the spine than through all of the organs.* This is why the SEF chart shows the kidneys on the inside of the foot with an adrenal gland atop each kidney.

The adrenal glands have two parts: an outer cortex and the inner medulla. All of the hormones secreted by the adrenal glands are under the direction of adrenocorticotropic hormone secreted by the pituitary gland in the brain. The adrenal cortex produces sex hormones like testosterone and estrogen. It also secretes the hormones cortisol and corticosterone (these are anti-inflammatory), which regulate blood pressure, blood sugar, and protein breakdown as well as support muscle function. DHEA, another hormone secreted by the cortex, has been found to affect the heart, body weight, immune and nervous systems, and bones. The medulla produces epinephrine and norepinephrine, which are commonly known as stress hormones because they are secreted during fear and stress (fight or flight).

These hormones energize the muscles of the circulatory (heart) and digestive systems. Excessive stimulation of this system over time can lead to exhaustion.

LOCATE AND WORK THE ADRENAL GLAND

The two adrenal glands are marked #5 on the SEF Chart. To locate the adrenal gland, first identify the waistline. Walk the thumb along the inside of the spine near the waistline while feeling for the kidney-shaped energy field. After locating the kidney, walk up the kidney field toward the toes with your thumb using very small bites until you get to the top of the field where the adrenal gland sits. When you get there, pause and position the inner aspect of your thumb directly over the point of maximum intensity and ring the bell. Visualize the colors and petals of the chakra along with the adrenal gland bathed in violet fire. You might also choose to visualize healthy adrenal glands using pictures from an anatomy and physiology book. The adrenal gland points are typically very tender. Be sure to use spirals and calming holds as needed to move the energy released from the field when sending the signal.

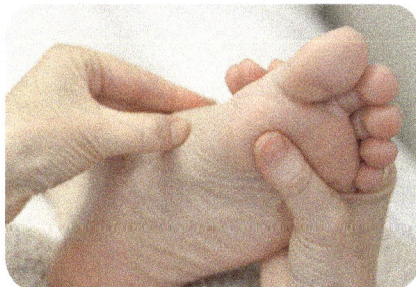

2-5 ADRENALS/SOLAR PLEXUS CHAKRA

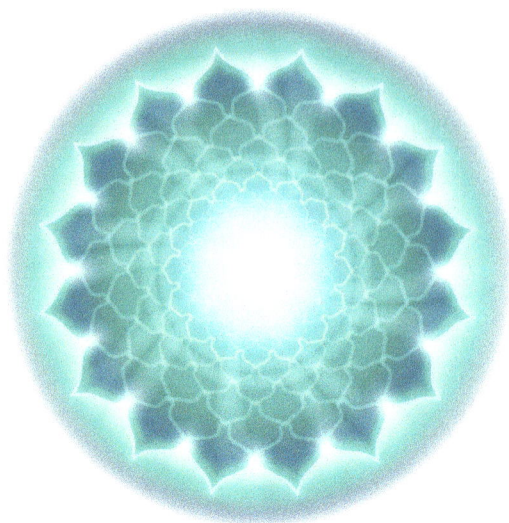

THIRD EYE

CHAKRA

The vibration of the third eye chakra is vision. The color is emerald green. The chakra has 96 petals. The difference between seeing through the third eye and seeing through our two physical eyes is that the third-eye vision center we see is discriminatory. Thus, we are able to perceive what can be as the blueprint of life manifests within and before us rather than what may actually be before us. It is this ability of the third eye that allows us to hold the balance for descent of wholeness even when someone is ill with disease or dying. Disease is human creation. Seeing people in terms of their disease is an expression of vision at the level of the human being. Third-eye vision offers a way of seeing from the dimension of the Creator of the blueprint. From this perspective come new ideas, remedies, and solutions to any and all of that which ails humanity. Vision with the third eye is a gift, which may manifest as clairvoyance. But many who practice SEF and are not clairvoyant can develop perception with their inner vision. Parents, for example, use their inner vision when they look at their newborn child and perceive that child in the future having manifested all of the talents and treasures s/he brought to create a meaningful life.

In the healing arts, it is important to discuss intuition, vision, and psychic energy. There is a nurse scientist who refers to intuition as "rapid critical thinking."[13] I think that that is so, but there is also a deep spiritual process of development of intuition that is involved. A person cannot simply become intuitive by being a critical thinker who speeds up the process by knowing his or her craft and practicing the way a musician learns to play an instrument or a dancer learns to dance. Intuitive ability such as vision involves another element, which Christians call "Grace" and others refer to as "gifts" or "spiritual attainment." Every musician, dancer, and artist realizes that they can mentally learn their art form and practice, even exert will in the quest to achieve perfection, but there comes a point when one really does not know if or when spiritual attainment or mastery will be achieved. So we "work while we have the light" of life force in our bodies. The ancient wisdom tradition is that this work is to serve humanity. This is the focus for spiritual development and the key to developing attainment rather than dabbling in psychic thralldom and mistaking it for vision.

True spiritual vision cannot and will not be enslaved or forced by the mind. The mind is a trickster, often casting illusion into the field of human perception. Ideas and mental impressions come and go like the wind. The mind alone should not dictate SEF work. It is a holistic model of care that includes accessing the spiritual, emotional, physical, and essential elements of Self through the senses, and provides a check and balance to the winds of the mind and mental body. Nature

---

13   (Benner, 2001)

scientist Johann Wolfgang von Goethe once said that "the senses do not deceive; the judgment deceives."[14] Educating the mind through study and skill development leads to greater understanding of the hologram, human anatomy and physiology, and the healing arts, which can lead to improved "seeing," analysis, and judgment of health patterns. Education and study provide the platform for the rooting of intuition.

Intuition is the "form in which thought-content first arises."[15] In contrast to perception, which is an externalized orientation, thought-content comes from within us. Philosopher and nature-scientist Rudolf Steiner describes intuition as being connected to thinking as "observation is to perception. Intuition and observation are the sources of our knowledge."[16] Intuition is important in making connection with and ultimately knowing our environment and those whom we seek to help with SEF. However, intuitive promptings *without* "roots" anchored in the mental body, thought, and intellect can lead to disturbances in the self of the SEF Provider and inappropriate care of the Partner that reach beyond one's skill and spiritual attainment to perceive the feet clearly. Education of the mental body and continued study is the antidote that can keep the trickster in check.

Dr. Laurence and Mrs. Phoebe Bendit refer to intuition without rooting in the mental body as a "negative psychic state."[17] Dr. Bendit was a Jungian psychiatrist and his wife, Phoebe, a clairvoyant. Psychic sense is similar to the other five senses in that it can be dull or acute. Negative psychism is uncontrolled, undifferentiated, and primitive. A person in a negative psychic state cannot differentiate the products of his own

---

14 (Goethe & Naydler, 1996)
15 (Steiner, 1995, p. 88)
16 (Steiner, 1995)
17 (Bendit & Bendit, 1958, p. 109)

mind from that which is external to it. Reactions are most often uncon-scious. The Bendits locate the mechanism of action of the negative psychic state in the coeliac plexus, which is in the center of the body. In SEF, this is referred to as the solar plexus. The openness of the negative psychic state can be observed as leading to unchecked projection of thought onto clients ("I know more about you than you know about yourself"), spiritual boundary violations, and physical problems.

The positive psychic state, however, is controlled and consciously directed by a person. The mechanism of action of the positive psychic state occurs in the head and the heart. It develops with maturity as the person learns to exhibit greater and greater discernment and discrimination, and make deliberate choices in response to intuitive impressions. The Bendits explain that society is still very much under the influence of primitive "urges" and "only partly governed by the conscious mind."[18] The refinement of the positive psychic state informed by intuition begins when the intellect is engaged and applied in analyzing and making conscious choices about the intuitive or psychic promptings. In the case of SEF, in which energy fields are routinely encountered, all intuitive promptings of the Provider and the Partner about patterns in the feet would be informed and checked against the awareness born of experience and knowledge. Patterns assessed in the feet during SEF should not be interpreted solely on intuitive or psychic hunches. This is not a holistic approach and the risk is too great. As stated above, the focus is to serve humanity. Wash the Partner's feet, anoint them and give them a good SEF treatment. SEF is not a platform for the wanton development of psychic states, mediumship, or the spiritualism that often pervades energy healing systems of care in current society.

---

18   Ibid.

The following are teachings on the subject from two renowned spiritual authors, Helena Roerich and Manly P. Hall (as cited by H. Roerich).

> *It is the greatest mistake to regard mediumistic faculties as spiritual achievements ... spirituality is always accompanied by balance and inborn wisdom. It will probably be wise at this point to describe the difference between a medium and a clairvoyant. To the average person there is no difference, but to the mystic these two phases of spiritual sight are separated by the entire span of human evolution. A clairvoyant is one who has raised the spinal serpent into the brain and by his growth earned the right of perceiving the invisible worlds with the aid of the third eye, or pineal gland....Clairvoyants are not born; they are made. Mediums are not made; they are born. The clairvoyant can become such only after years, sometimes lives, of self-preparation; on the other hand, the medium, ... may secure results in a few days. But of course one should add here that the medium is limited to the lower strata of the Subtle World.[19] What ignorance is displayed in thinking that the highest and subtlest can be achieved by purely mechanical methods! You are quite right when you say that people, in striving for spiritual development (which to them so often means the achievement of psychic powers), forget that without service to the General Good this development will be one-sided and unstable. Our inner fires are kindled only through contact with people. Only thus can we test ourselves; only thus shall we be able to sharpen and temper the blade of our spirit.[20]*

The third eye chakra is associated with the pineal gland in the brain. The pineal gland is the shape of a pinecone and contains nerve cells similar to those in the retina of the eye. It is typically quite small, the size of a grain of wheat. "It is a relic of the third eye, which was

---

19   (Roerich, 1967, pp. 51, 124-125)
20   (Roerich, 1967, p. 27)

an early organ for the purpose of sensing light and shadows. We may properly refer to it as an organ of inner world contact. It secretes an etheric light substance in a manner resembling the pinecone's exudation of resin."[21] This gland is the bridge between a higher plane of consciousness and the physical plane of expression.[22]

The pineal gland works with the pituitary gland as an organ of transmutation and regeneration. It works with the thymus gland in early life to hold sex in abeyance and retains some mechanism for the action of light upon the pigment of the skin. It secretes melatonin, the hormone responsible for the regulation of sleep and the biological clock.

LOCATE AND WORK THE PINEAL GLAND

The pineal gland is marked #6 on the SEF Chart. To locate the pineal gland, you will be working the great toe [zone 1]. Hold and support the foot with your inside hand and stabilize the great toe. Using the outside thumb and forefinger, place the upper outer contact point of your thumb on the inner aspect of the toenail for the great toe. Roll your thumb toward the toe and down very slightly and then ring the bell. Visualize the colors and petals of the chakra along with the pineal gland bathed in violet fire. You might also choose to visualize a healthy pineal gland using pictures from an anatomy and physiology book. The pineal gland points are located on both feet. Be sure to use spirals and calming holds as needed to move the energy released from the field when sending the signal. Circle the great toe while stabilizing it at the base. This action is similar to rotating the head 360 degrees on the neck. Notice as you are performing the 360-degree toe circling in which degree(s) you feel a free flow of energy and which are tense, stiff, and therefore blocked.

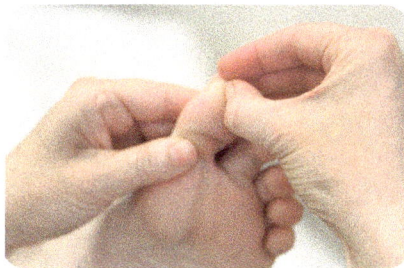

2-6 PINEAL/THIRD EYE CHAKRA

---

21   (Heline, 1991 (originally published 1937), p. 249)
22   (Kapp, 1958, p. 25)

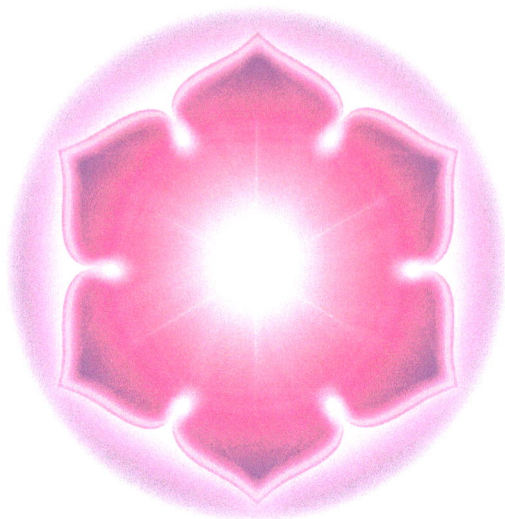

SEAT-OF-THE-SOUL
CHAKRA

The vibration of the Seat-of-the-Soul chakra is freedom, mercy, and joy. The color is violet. The chakra has six petals representing the ascending and descending triangles that are intertwined and form a six-pointed star. These petals are the integration of spirit and matter in the alchemy of the soul as it strives for freedom through transmutation of all karmic bonds that prevent the soul from being all it is meant to be. Through the freedom center, we experience the sweetness of life, a gift from the Creator that is the ultimate opportunity to balance karma and fulfill dharma or righteousness—the "right-useness" of God's gift of life. Children first receive this opportunity as they are faced with their choice between their desire to play and their desire to learn and study. "The adult who lives without cultivating and employing his innate powers of wisdom and spiritual discrimination finds inexorably that the kingdom of the body and mind is being overrun by the insurgents of misery-making wrong desires, destructive habits, failure, ignorance, disease, and unhappiness."[23] This is why visualization of the violet fire, which vibrates in harmony with the Seat-of-the-Soul chakra, is a major focus of SEF, in which the understanding is given that changes can be made to the focus of desires, health habits, and any disease process that manifests as a health pattern. The action to change and, more so, to actually *transmute* the energy of *what has been* into the blueprint of *what is* (whole) at the etheric level occurs in the vibration of the Seat-of-the-Soul chakra.

The Seat-of-the-Soul chakra is associated with the pancreas. The pancreas energy field covers zones 1-4 in the Partner's left foot and 1-2 zones in the right. The right side of the pancreas is the "head" and the left side extending up to the spleen is referred to as the "tail." The spleen is the largest ductless gland in the body. It lies between the stomach and the diaphragm muscle under the ribs. The spleen produces red and white blood corpuscles that are part of the immune response. It also stores iron in the blood and aids in digestion. The spleen can be likened to a solar energy station in the body as it channels the etheric energy that nourishes the nervous system. The pancreas aids in digestion and secretes the hormones insulin and glucagon, which help to regulate blood glucose and are involved in metabolism. Insulin is secreted by the beta cells of the pancreas in response to elevated blood glucose levels. The alpha cells secrete glucagon. Its presence allows for the absorption of sugar into the cells. The enzymes in the pancreas help to break down fats, proteins, carbohydrates, and acids in the duodenum.

---

23   (Yogananda, 1995, p. 8)

LOCATE AND WORK THE PANCREAS

The pancreas is marked #7 on the SEF Chart. To locate the pancreas, you will be working both feet. Start by locating the waistline on the Partner's right foot. Then support their right foot with your left hand while you walk the pancreas with your right thumb. Flex or bend the toes back slightly as you watch for the tendon in the sole of the foot to come out. The tendon is the border of the first zone. Walk from the inside of the sole of the foot at the waistline up to the tendon. You are walking the head of the pancreas on this foot. On the Partner's left foot, you will be walking the tail of the pancreas that extends from the first up to the fifth zone where it attaches to the spleen #25. Thumb walk from zone 1 using small bites. Be sure to flex the toes to visualize the tendon. On this foot, you will jump over the tendon when you are thumb walking because working the tendon can cause excessive discomfort to your Partner. Because the pancreas touches the spleen, it is very simple to work the spleen after the pancreas. Work the spleen #25 with thumb walking or a spiral action with the knuckle of your middle finger. This knuckle technique is used extensively and some-times exclusively in Ersdal Foot Zone Therapy treatments. I typically use it when seeking to reach organs, such as the spleen and gallbladder, that reside at a deeper level (in the hologram) of the body. Make a gentle fist and extend the central knuckle of the middle finger. The tip of the knuckle can be very effective for moving energy in the spleen, which extends across the fifth zone above the waistline and below the ball of the left foot. Visualize the colors and petals of the Seat-of-the-Soul chakra along with the pancreas bathed in violet fire. You might also choose to visualize a healthy pancreas and spleen using pictures from an anatomy and physiology book. The pancreas points are located on both feet. Be sure to use spirals and calming holds as needed to move the energy released from the field when sending the signal.

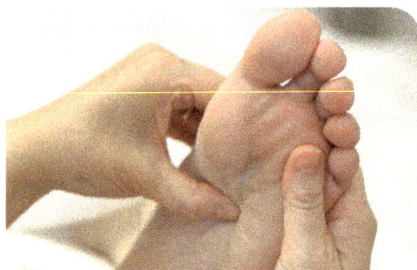

2-7 PANCREAS/SEAT OF THE SOUL

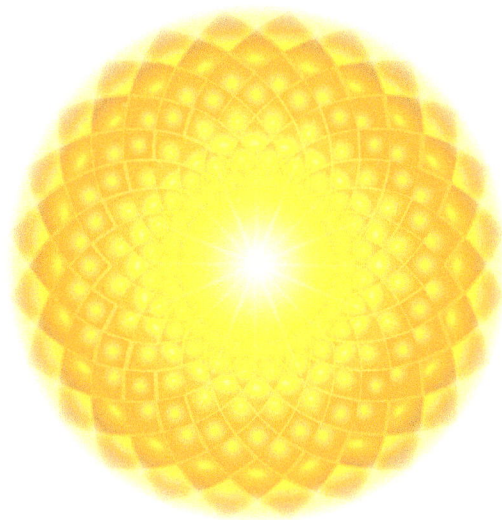

CROWN

CHAKRA

The vibration of the crown chakra is wisdom. The color is golden yellow. The chakra has 972 petals, but is referred to as the "thousand-petaled lotus." Through the wisdom center, we focus on the consciousness of God the Creator. The enlightenment of the Buddha, the Christ, and the Divine Mother is experienced in the crown as a deep sense of knowing all things without being taught. We see the spiral of knowledge descend in nature as a number arrangement associated with the Fibonacci sequence [24] and, therefore, the harmony of the golden ratio in the spiral

---

24   The golden ratio (also known as the golden mean or by its Greek name [and symbol], phi [Φ]), the mathematical proportion numerically approximated 1.618034…ad infinitum, is, as nature demonstrates, the foundation of organic harmony, beauty, and balance. Many artists, philosophers, scientists, mathematicians, and architects consider the golden ratio an essential component of beauty if not life itself. Ancient Egyptians knew the importance of phi in nature and built the pyramids that still stand today. Leonardo Fibonacci, a thirteenth-century mathematician, found the numerical sequence generated by the golden ratio. The sequence of numbers consists of terms that are the sum of the two preceding terms (1, 1, 2, 3, 5, 8, 13 …).

pattern of the pinecone, the head of the sunflower, the beehive, and in the human inner ear. Goethe wrote, "Beauty is a manifestation of secret natural laws, which otherwise would have been hidden from us forever." In SEF, the spiraling action we make with our hands within the context (vibration) of the hologram can energetically simulate the rhythm or harmony of that which is within our own DNA and that of our Partner as well as nature herself. In SEF, we meditate in the crown chakra on channeling the harmony of the spheres as the geometry of divinity (G-O-D). We invoke the full manifestation of wisdom of nature as we meditate upon her shape in objects found in nature and the human body while sending signals through the hologram in the feet to the blueprint of wholeness. This action is akin to the harmony of the buzzing of a honeybee and humming of the hummingbird. And so, as we activate the crown chakra through its glandular counterpart—the pituitary, we hum, making sure to allow for the resonation of the "m" as in mother to manifest the healing action of the beauty of the crown chakra. In the Vedic tradition, the sounding of the AUM also accomplishes this action with A representing Alpha and M, Omega. A complete sounding of the AUM (which takes mastery) potentiates the activation of the wholeness current in SEF—Alpha to Omega, the beginning and the ending.

The pituitary gland is the master gland, the energetic catalyst and, therefore, the teacher within as the wisdom of the crown chakra suggests. The wisdom of the body is contained within a gland the size of a pea. That tells something of the power of the Creator in nature. It is small yet not so simple to understand, except perhaps through spiritual retreat into the inner recesses of the mind-body continuum. The pituitary gland directs the action of mind-body processes. For example, it oversees the release of hormones that govern the neuropeptide releases related to emotional states that strengthen immune response.[25]

---

25   (Pert, 1997)

The anterior pituitary orchestrates the body's glands. It also secretes prolactin, the hormone that stimulates and sustains milk production after birth and governs sexual development. The posterior pituitary secretes antidiuretic hormone and oxytocin regulates fluid balance in the body, blood pressure, the gastrointestinal tract (and peristaltic, or wave-like action, through the system), fat, and sugar metabolism. There is more vitamin E in the pituitary than any other gland. Therefore, it requires vitamin E to function well. The pituitary also requires adequate amounts of vitamin B, manganese, and copper to function well.

LOCATE AND WORK THE PITUITARY

The pituitary gland is marked #8 on the SEF Chart. To locate the pituitary, you will be working the great toe in zone 1 on both feet. Start by looking closely at the sole of the great toe. Imagine the bottom of the toe above the neck area drawn into four quadrants. Typically on the lower inside quadrant (the side next to the second toe), there will be a noticeable "tent" of skin at the center of the spiraling toe print on the skin. The pituitary and crown chakra sit beneath this tent.

To ring the bell of the pituitary, locate the tent through visual inspection and then begin your thumb walking with very small bites superficially until you feel the surge of energy of the crown. Support the toe with your outside hand while walking the toe area with the inside thumb. When on the crown, ring the bell to send the signal. It is key to practice so that you can support the toe without sending signals—that is, not pressing with the supporting hand. Visualize the colors and petals of the crown chakra along with the pituitary gland bathed in violet fire. You might also choose to visualize a healthy pituitary using pictures from an anatomy and physiology book. The pituitary points are located on both feet. Be sure to use spirals and calming holds as needed to move the energy released from the field when sending the signal.

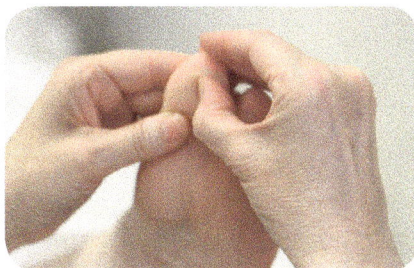

2-8 PITUITARY/CROWN CHAKRA

BASE-OF-THE-SPINE

CHAKRA

The vibration of the Base-of-the-Spine chakra is purity. The color is white,[26] the color of the sun on newly fallen snow. The base chakra has four petals, foundational for physical incarnation represented in the elements of all matter: fire, air, water, and earth. Just as the 4/4 rhythm of a march or what is known as "common time" in music and dance evokes stability, strength, and harmony, so too do the four petals of the base chakra. The purity center is the focal point for the light of Mother as she is manifest in every human form. The body is Mother and the base chakra is the essence and consciousness of the light of Mother. "It is from this point that man rises for the reunion of Mother with the Father in the crown, which brings forth the Christ in

---

26   See section, Golden Understanding, later in the chapter for further explanation of the importance of the white chakra.

the center of the heart."[27] In the East, this light rising along the spine is referred to as the "kundalini." It is the sacred fire of Mother light that enables man and woman to embody not just physically but also mentally, emotionally, and spiritually—that is, to be incarnated in the fullest expression of human life.

Human life is initiated with energy flow through the gonads or sex glands of man and woman toward the fulfillment of the highest form of creative act. Gonad is the Greek word for seed and refers to the testes in men and the ovaries in women. The ovaries in a woman produce the egg, which travels through the fallopian tubes to the uterus or womb where the egg will implant and develop if fertilized into a human being. The ovaries also produce substances that make a woman feminine. The reproductive system of a woman includes the breasts as well. The male testes produce semen, which carries the sperm from the prostate gland into the woman where it may fertilize the ovum. "The internal secretion of the cortex of the testes is the male energizing force and that which makes him really male."[28] All of the organs of the female and male reproductive systems rely on hormone secretions from other glands to catalyze their functions.

The functions of the gonads have a higher and a lower state of life. In astrological science, the gonads "respond to Virgo-Pisces in higher life and to Taurus-Scorpio in lower. The masses respond to the lower sense impulses of Scorpio and Taurus; the regenerate respond to the purity of Virgo and the chaste Neptunian ray of Pisces. The gonadic force must be lifted in order to unite with the pineal gland and pituitary body in the intricate processes of the Mystic Marriage."[29] From these glands that exude generative energy, a small amount

---

27 (Kul & Prophet, 1980, p. Plate 8)
28 (Kapp, 1958, p. 35)
29 (Heline, 1991 (originally published 1937), p. 271)

of oil is excreted. The oil increases in potency and volume as the person's emotions become more pure in acts of service to humanity in commemoration of the Mystic Marriage—the union of vision (Pineal) and higher consciousness (Pituitary), spirit and matter. The parable of the Wise virgins in the Bible demonstrates the teaching of those who garner the light in the base chakra, for example, by honoring the sacredness of the oil of the seed of life within man and woman. They have access to the Bridegroom and the light that is available for regenerative processes and healing. That light is the white light of the Mother, or *kundalini*, that is stored in the Base-of-the-Spine chakra, which then rises to the crown.

Yogananda describes the "awakened" kundalini as a "power flowing from the coccyx to Spirit" that is "fire" or "life energy."[30] "Under King Soul, the creative 'Mother Nature' in the coccyx is calm and controlled, bringing health, beauty, and peace to the kingdom. At the command of the yogi in deep meditation, this creative force turns inward and flows back to its source in the thousand-petaled lotus, revealing the resplendent inner world of the divine forces and consciousness of the soul and Spirit."[31] SEF is a meditation practice and active service rooted in understanding congruent with many spiritual traditions. SEF is a practice of focused spiritual attention on the white-fire core as Mother or Mater (Matter) in every chakra.

---

30   (Yogananda, 1995, p. 741)
31   (Yogananda, 1995, p. 18)

LOCATE AND WORK THE GONADS

The gonads (reproductive system) are marked #9 and #10 on the SEF Chart. They are located on both feet. The breast area will be discussed in the next chapter in the section on the lymphatic system. To locate the gonads in men and women, you will be working the sides of the heel area on both feet below the ankle. To ring the bell for the gonads, hold the points on either side of the heel with one hand. With your palm up facing you, cradle your middle finger and thumb around the back of the heel and wrap the tip of those fingers in to press #9 (inside – middle finger) and #10 (outside – thumb). Try circling the foot between the thumb and middle finger, ringing the bell on one side and then the other while visualizing the rising of the Mother light energy along the spine like a winged caduceus. There is an energetic connection between the two points. When your location is correct, you will feel a surge of energy drawing the tips of your middle finger and thumb toward each other like a magnet. Visualize the white color and four petals of the base-of-the-spine chakra along with the pituitary gland bathed in violet fire. You might also choose to visualize a healthy uterus, fallopian tubes, and ovaries in a woman or healthy testes and prostate in a man using pictures from an anatomy and physiology book. These points are often close to the surface and sensitive so be sure to use spirals and calming holds as needed to move the energy released from the field when sending the signal. After working the energy field for the base-of-the-spine chakra/gonads, visualize drawing the released light up to the third eye as you walk the spine from the sacrum to the head.

Do this by rotating the hand that is cradling the heel so that your fingers lay flat across the top of the ankle. Allow your thumb to follow the rotation from point #10 to the sacrum and begin the spine walk. After the spine walk, do a spine stretch (See Chapter 1).

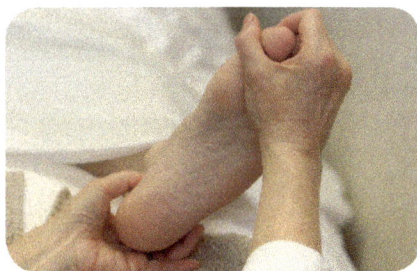

2-9 GONADS/BASE-OF-THE-SPINE CHAKRA

GLAND In spiraling order	CHAKRA	COLOR	PETALS*
Thymus	Heart - Love	Pink	12
Thyroid	Throat - Power	Blue	16
Adrenals	Solar Plexus - Peace	Purple and Gold	10
Pineal	Third Eye-Vision	Emerald Green	96
Pancreas	Seat-of-the-Soul— Freedom/Mercy	Violet	6
Pituitary	Crown-Wisdom	Golden Yellow	972
Gonads	Base — Foundation/ Materialization	White	4

*Note: The numbers of petals are listed here for educational purposes. The energy or vibration of the chakras, and the number of petals representing that vibration, do change.

2-10   CHAKRA CHART

GOLDEN UNDERSTANDING

The mystical union as the ultimate unity of spirit and matter occurs gradually, as Spirit becomes matter and matter becomes Spirit once again. This is a process of evolution as the self (with a lower case s) of the lower nature is realized into the Self (with a capital S) of one's higher nature in God as a co-Creator in life. This process has been referred to throughout time as the *alchemy* of personal transformation. Carl Jung stated in his book *Alchemical Studies* that the alchemists of old did not seek to make ordinary gold but were working with "philosophical gold."[32] Because SEF taps into the blueprint of wholeness, we are working with the gold of the spirit also. SEF treatments are life transforming through spiritual practice and service to others. This is why the visualization of the unique vibration (color and number of petals) of the chakras becomes critical to the alchemical process of the transformation of the self of Provider and Partner alike.

There are religious traditions that represent the Base-of-the-Spine—or what is often referred to as the "root" chakra—in different shades of red and orange. The colors of the Base-of-the-Spine chakra and all of the major chakras are depicted in the SEF book and chart as they appear at the level of the etheric blueprint. Light as energy in vibration or movement manifests as color (and also sound). In SEF, the vibration of the energy of Mother is understood as the color white.

Red and white are both alchemical colors, with red signifying the sun and white the moon.[33] But one must take the greatest care in visualizing red in association with the Base-of-the-Spine chakra so as to achieve a vibration that will raise the process to a level of healing

---

32   (Jung, 1968b, p. 243)
33   (Jung, 1968a, p. 339)

and wholeness that is separate from the vibration of disease and decay. For example, Blavatsky, a Buddhist scholar, taught that the "transcendent red or golden orange of the sun must not be confused with the scarlet kama-rupan redness."[34] Kama-rupa is a Sanskrit word referring to man's passionate nature. Instead, during an SEF treatment, the Base-of-the-Spine chakra should not be visualized in a way that resonates with the lower passionate nature but as its highest vibration that will lift the spirits of the Partner and create a magnet for the light of Mother as beauty and healing. That vibration is symbolized in the white of the moon or Mother. While the alchemy of the color of the sun—the red-orange of Father—might be appropriate for some of great spiritual attainment, the color is too close to the vibration that is not conducive to the healing energy held in the SEF Tau Spiral chakra meditation.

Many depictions of the Base-of-the-Spine chakra utilize the red color that resonates with the lower level of man's state of consciousness on the planet rather than with that of the etheric pattern of wholeness. The red vibration around the Base-of-the-Spine chakra— even as it may appear in an advanced embodied "adept" or sage—can actually be an accumulation of anger (redness in the face) from people on the planet. The adept has the ability and vision to transmute the energies associated with the red color through service and meditation. But those who do not have the attainment in the healing arts could sit with the anger, which in some patterns is even being expressed as hatred of the Mother, as a result of their own choices and possibly as a result of the energy they have agreed to take on in the alchemical process of transmutation.

Knowledge of the human body's capacity to transmute energy

---

34   As cited in (Cranston, 1993, p. 42)

is not new. The origin of the ancient wisdom traditions is the spiritual path of alchemy. Those who have applied these principles in the healing arts recognize the spiritual path of alchemy as taught by Hermes Trismegistus, the mythical figure whom the Greeks considered a messenger of the gods and the Egyptians equated with Thoth, the god of knowledge, who stated that matter was the "vehicle of becoming."[35] The focus of the healing arts, such as SEF, is the promotion of embodiment of Self as matter in which it becomes abundantly clear that God the Creator is the doer rather than the ego of the SEF Provider. Both the Provider and the Partner are given the opportunity in the spiritual service of SEF to transmute and transform self and *become* Self.

Light is drawn into the chakras. Through the act of flow, that light then nourishes all other centers, organs, and systems in the matter world of the person. There is a light or fire released in the process that is then sent back to the source, raising consciousness and connecting all with the realm of Spirit once again. This is the cycle of *energy flow* that, once established, is then sent from the chakras to the other body systems. The hands move to activate a wholeness current in each of those other systems. The next chapter describes the step-by-step treatment of the remaining body systems.

Bendit, P., & Bendit, L. (1958). *Our Psychic Sense: A Clairvoyant and A Psychiatrist Explain How it Works.* London: Quest Books.

Benner, P. (2001). *From Novice to Expert: Excellence and Power in Clinical Nursing Practice.* New Jersey: Prentice-Hall.

Bible - King James Version. (1972). United States: Thomas Nelson, Publishers.

Blavatsky, H. (1888). *The Secret Doctrine: The Synthesis of Science, Religion, and Philosophy.* London: The Theosophical Publishing Co.

Cranston, S. (1993). *HPB: The Extraordinary Life and Influence of Helena Blavatsky Founder of the Modern Theosophical Movement.* New York: G.P. Putnam's Sons.

Diamond, J. (1979). *Behavioral Kinesiology: How to Activate Your Thymus and Increase Your Life Energy.* New York: Harper & Row.

Goethe, J. W., & Naydler, J. (1996). *Goethe on Science.* Edinburgh: Floris Books.

Heline, C. (1991 (originally published 1937)). *Occult Anatomy and the Bible.* Los Angeles: New Age Press.

Jung, C. G. (1968a). *Alchemical Studies* (Vol. XIII). Princeton, NJ: Princeton University Press.

Jung, C. G. (1968b). *Psychology and Alchemy* (Vol. XII). Princeton, NJ: Princeton University Press.

Kapit, W., & Elson, L. M. (2001). *The Anatomy Coloring Book* (3rd ed.). San Francisco: Benjamin Cummings.

Kapp, M. (1958). *Glands - Our Invisible Guardians* (Vol. XVIII, Rosicrucian Library). San Jose, California: Supreme Grand Lodge of AMORC.

Kul, D., & Prophet, E. C. (1980). *Intermediate Studies of the Human Aura.* Los Angeles, California: Summit University Press.

Pert, C. (1997). *Molecules of Emotion.* New York: Scribner.

Roerich, H. (1967). *Letters of Helena Roerich 1935-1939.* New York: Agni Yoga Society.

Steiner, R. (1995). *Intuitive Thinking as a Spiritual Path.* Dornach, Switzerland: Anthroposophic Press.

Yogananda, P. (1995). *The Bhagavad Gita.* Los Angeles: Self-Realization Fellowship.

Yukteswar, S. S. (1990 (Originally published 1949)). *The Holy Science.* Los Angeles, California: Self Realization Fellowship.

CHAPTER THREE

Completing the Basic Treatment Step by Step

Once the preparation steps and the Tau Spiral chakra meditation are completed, the channels for the flow of energy and light are then open for the descent of the blueprint. The rest of the basic treatment is focused on sending signals for each of the organ systems. The thumb, fingers, and both hands are used to deliver a wholeness current to move the energy in all fields that may be blocked.

Blocks of energy are felt in the anatomic systems in different ways because the physiology and energy flow through the systems is unique to each system. For example, the flow through the colon follows a very specific direction through a single "tube" so that waste matter can be excreted from the body. The lymphatic system also has an excreting function in the body, but there are multiple vessels that are active in the process.

An overview of a brief anatomy and physiology of each of the systems discussed in this chapter will be provided with an emphasis on the specific energy flow patterns unique to that system. Learning the interface between the physiology of a system, the flow, the blueprint, and SEF treatment is an ongoing process. Follow the earlier directions for recognizing blocks in energy flow through placement, pain, and pattern. Additional aspects of the anatomy and physiology of a system and its connection to the work will be found when caring for Partners, each of whom is a unique person. The information that is presented here is essential to a basic SEF treatment and serves only as a platform for further inspiration and development in the application of the SEF technique for each unique person.

The techniques used in step-by-step working of the systems are the same as those previously used in the preparations for the basic treatment and in the treatment of the glandular system and chakras during the Tau Spiral meditation. Although human anatomy is basically the same from person to person, the energy patterns in each pair of feet are unique. There are differences in anatomy caused by injury, illness, or birth defect. In SEF, the person is treated according to the divine blueprint of wholeness. Therefore, if a person has had, for example, their appendix removed, the energy field for the appendix in the foot can still be treated. Consideration of this fundamental maxim of practice can lead to greater understanding of holographic science when applied in the care of people. The goal is to move the energy, but not by brute force. Visualize the healthy, whole organs; transmute energy blockages with violet fire; ensure proper landmark and organ placement before sending signals; and stay on a point only long enough to "ring the bell" to make an energetic connection with the field.

As a momentum in SEF work is developed, the patterns of wholeness representing "normal" energy flow in all human beings' organ systems becomes more apparent. Take care to not develop expectations of normality and project them on to a Partner. This can lead to negative thoughts that pathologize another's pattern. Pathologize means to associate behaviors with disease or illness. For example, pregnancy and aging are both "normal" parts of life that may be pathologized or perceived at times as illness.

SEF practice and preparation includes fostering a state of mind-fulness that is defined by openness to the possibility of the emergence of a new "normal" at any time. The SEF Provider's overall process of interpretation that occurs when working the organ systems includes comparing what is felt in the feet to what is known about normal anatomy and physiology, but the Provider suspends judgment about any deviations from normal. When there is a thought that something is amiss in the feet, the first step is to presume that hand placement is incorrect. This is part of the ethic of SEF work. Each of the organ and system descriptions that follow includes common areas for caution related to working with energy blockages and deviations from normal anatomy and physiology. It is best to work all of the systems on one foot first and then the other. Because of the anatomical structure of the large intestine, it is best to begin the work on the gastrointestinal system on the Partner's right foot and then work the left foot. In addition, the heart areas, a major part of the cardiovascular system [*See Figure 3-1*], have already been worked during the Tau Spiral meditation and the working of the thymus and thyroid glands. The aortic arch (#2) is worked on the *left* foot. Use a spiral knuckle technique to move the energy from the thymus (#3) up between the first and second zones and then in a curve over toward the area beneath the second toe. The blood vessels that make up the cardiovascular system are worked with the lymphatic system and when the foot is worked through with spiraling hand motions.

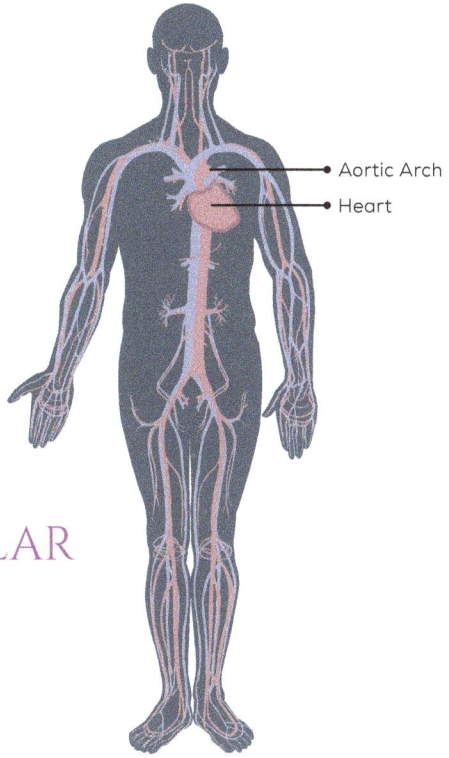

CARDIO-VASCULAR SYSTEM

Figure 3-1

- Aortic Arch
- Heart

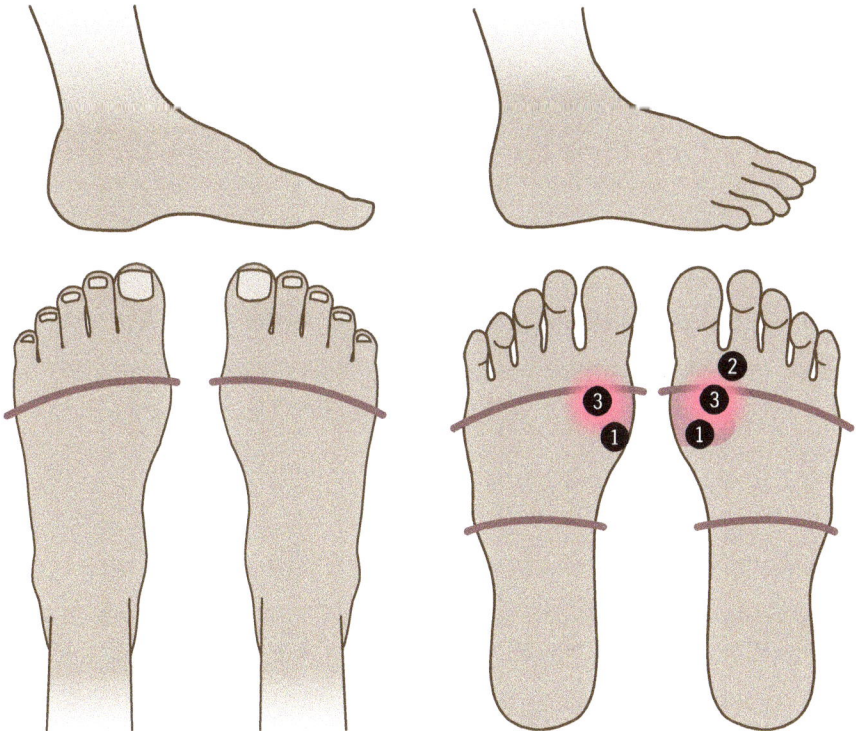

LYMPHATIC SYSTEM

The lymphatic system [*See Figure 3-2*] is an important part of the body's defense system. Upon the first touch of the feet, the lymphatic system is activated. This is due to the anatomical structure of the system, which comprises both superficial and deep vessels that form a network diffused throughout the body. Some areas of the body, such as the brain and spinal cord, do not have lymphatic vessels.

The body is largely fluid. Lymphatic vessels help veins function by draining many of the body tissues and thereby increasing the amount of fluid that returns to the heart. However, the heart does not pump the fluid in the lymph system. Muscle movement provides the force for movement in the lymph vessels. The lymphatic system is not closed like the cardiovascular system. Lymph vessels begin as tiny capillaries in body tissues and then merge with larger vessels that enter into fluid filtering stations called "nodes."

These nodes or gathering points are located in the cervical or neck area (#26), the axilla or armpits (#23), and the inguinal area or groin (#22). They benefit, in particular, from SEF work. Lymph nodes swell when infection is present in their area of drainage due to a proliferation of lymphocytes. They may also swell when cancer cells migrate or metastasize from lymph channels. Gentle massage and gargling (as in the case of throat infections) can assist in draining the lymph tissue and excretion of infectious "waste" that occurs as the result of the battle between the lymphocytes and microbes. The lymphatic system includes the spleen (#25), tonsils (#41), and breast (#24).

The action used to work these points is a pumping action that simulates muscle contraction and release. To work the cervical lymph nodes (#26), use the finger milking technique to pump the areas between each toe. [*See Chapter 1 Figure 1-4*] Visualize sending the fluid toward the lymph trunk in the center of the body for excretion as you

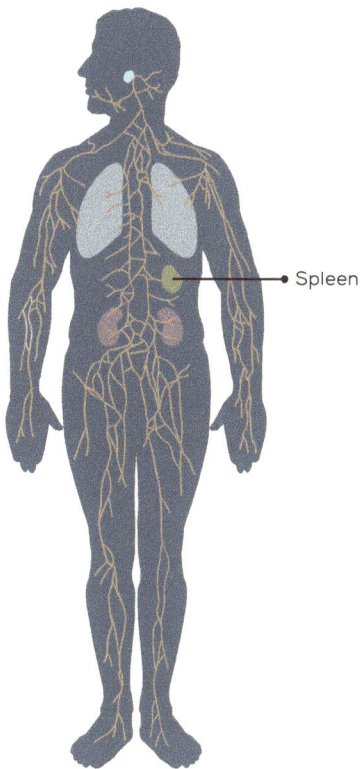

Spleen

LYMPHATIC SYSTEM

Figure 3-2

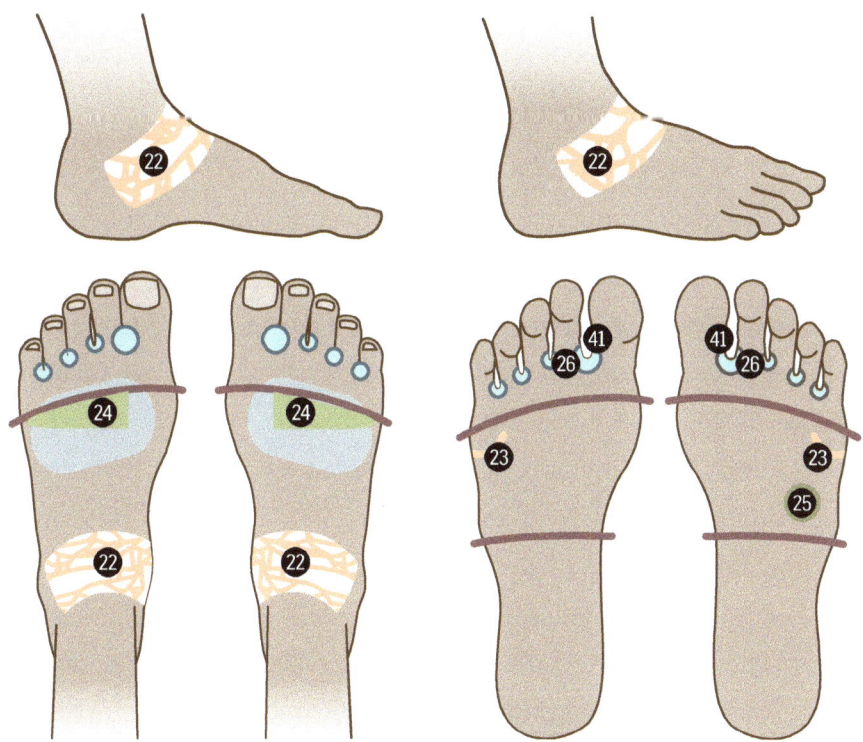

move from the neck to the axilla. Locate the shoulder on the foot. The shoulder is in the fifth zone at the end of the shoulder line. Run your fingers along the outside of the foot at the shoulder point and then along the outer edge of your actual shoulder joint. The roundness of the shoulder energy field feels very similar to the shoulder itself. The axillary lymph nodes run under the shoulder. Stabilize the foot as you thumb walk under the shoulder from the outer side of zone five to the beginning of zone four. Visualize the pumping action that you are simulating, and your thumb motion will take on a different quality or effort as discussed in Chapter 1.

After walking the axillary lymph nodes, switch your attention to your inside hand and the top of the foot to work the breast area. Your three middle fingers of the inside hand on the foot you are working should be nearly in position for working the breast after holding for the axillary lymph nodes. Gently stretch the toes toward you so that you can visualize the top of the foot. Line your fingertips along the tendon that runs along the top of the first zone (metatarsal for the great toe). This is the energy field for the sternum (See SEF Chart #15). The breast energy field extends from the sternum to the axillary area (outer side of the foot). It is the shape of a wing—wide near the sternum and forming a tip at the axilla. Because it is such a large area, use a finger wave technique to cross over and activate the energy field for the breast. [*See Chapter 1 Figure 1-16*]

Finish the lymphatic system by working through the whole foot with both hands [*See Chapter 1 Figure 1-17*] and then performing a finger wave across the top of the ankle from bone to bone. This technique moves the lymph of the groin area (#22). After the groin channels, use the knuckle technique and work the heel at the bottom of the foot. This pelvis area (See SEF Chart #21) includes large lymph vessels known as "trunks." The cisterna chyli, which typically sits across from the lumbar 1 – 2 vertebrae, is a central focus for the lymphatic system. A common draining trunk for most of the body's lymphatic vessels, the cisterna chyli is the beginning of the primary lymphatic vessel for the body known as the thoracic duct. The energy fields for the thoracic duct and cisterna chyli are activated when working the spine.

SPINE WALKING AND JOINTS

The spinal column is made up of seven cervical (#14), 12 thoracic (#13), five lumbar vertebrae (#12), and five sacral (#11) vertebrae that are fused into a single bone, and the tailbone or coccyx (#11). The same number on the wall chart designates the sacrum and coccyx because they are in such close proximity in the hologram of the foot. The spine may be "walked" from the sacrum/coccyx to the cervical 1 vertebra or base of the skull multiple times during a treatment. The spine provides protection for the spinal cord and the energy channels that run along the spine that are called in Sanskrit. the *ida* (positive current), *pingala* (negative current), and *sushumna* (main current). The seven cervical vertebrae represent the seven major celestial bodies—the Sun, Moon, Earth, Venus, Mercury, Saturn, and Jupiter. The 12 thoracic vertebrae relate to the 12 signs of the zodiac. The five bones of the lumbar spine relate to the five elements of all matter creation—Fire, Air, Water, Earth, and Ether. The five bones of the sacrum relate to the power of creation and the four bones of the coccyx the anchoring of the individual soul in the matter universe. These 33 bones of the spinal column constitute the physical altar for the creative energy in the body that resonates with the 33 degrees of mystical initiation, the seat of power where the forces of the head and the heart unite. Thirty-three is a mystic number identified and utilized in many traditions to signify

the years or degrees[1] required
for initiation on the spiritual
path toward enlightenment.
Thus, the spinal altar is itself
sacred as the place where the
light of life and beauty is
garnered. In SEF, each vertebra

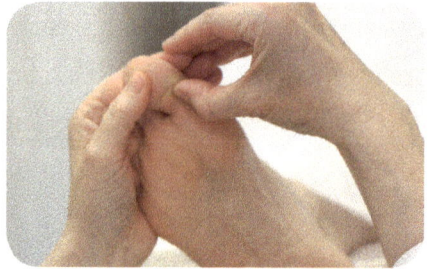

3-3 THUMB WALK THE NECK

is walked with reverence for the actual or potential life force manifest
within each bone segment. With each thrust of the thumb and ringing
of the bell, light is sent into the vertebrae to transmute all effluvia that
would impede the descent of light enlightenment.

If the spine were to represent the "trunk of the tree," that is the
body, the other major joints in the body are the limbs. The skeletal
structures—trunk and limbs—provide the scaffold for balance of the
entirety from head to toe. After walking the spine, work the head and
neck areas (#32 through #36). Stabilize the head area (toes) with your
outside hand. To work the neck, extend the great toe slightly so that
you can thumb walk the neck area in small lines—or what Oma and I
have always referred to as "stripes"—up into the ball of the toe (base of
skull). [*See Figure 3-3*] This technique works on any blockages not only
in muscles that may be tense in the neck, but also in any of the major
blood vessels that supply the brain with oxygen. Repeat with the four
remaining toes, walking in as tiny bites as possible from the base of the
toe to the ball of the toe. Although much of the great toe has already
been worked during the Tau Spiral, you may also choose to walk the
ball of the great toe in stripes so as to address each point of the head
and brain more specifically. It is more common to do this with Partners

---

1   In the Bible, David was initiated for 33 years before he could rule peacefully.
Jesus's mission on Earth was perfected in 33 years. In Masonic orders, there are 33
degrees of initiation.

JOINTS & HEAD AREAS

Figure 3-4

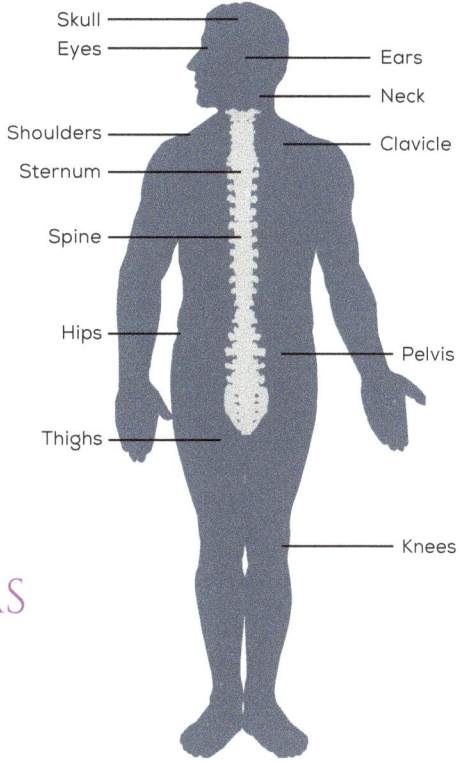

Skull — Ears
Eyes — Neck
Shoulders — Clavicle
Sternum
Spine
Hips — Pelvis
Thighs
Knees

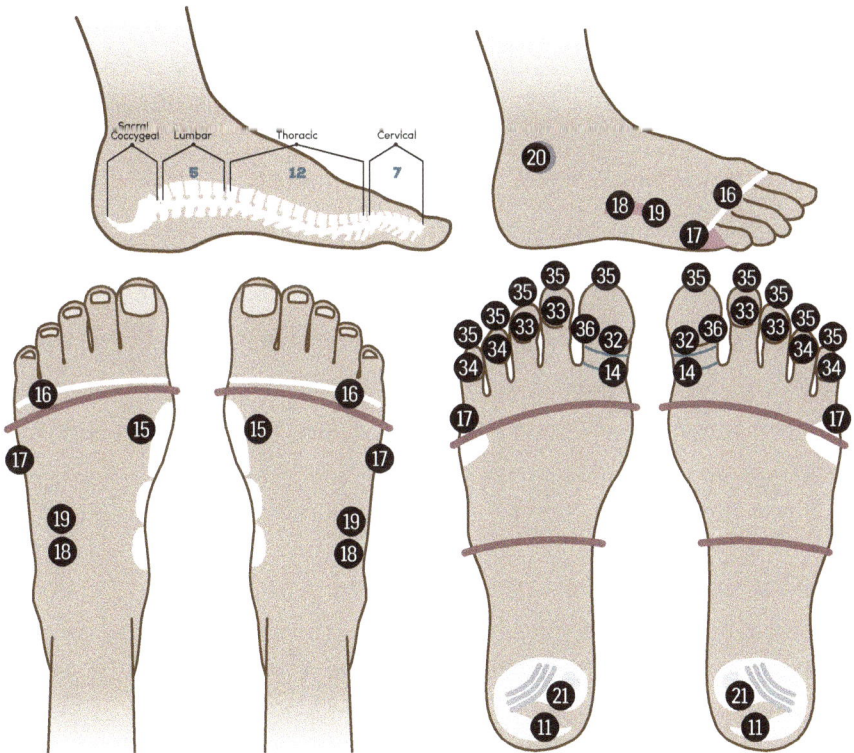

Sacral Coccygeal | Lumbar | Thoracic | Cervical
5 | 12 | 7

whose toes are larger. Remember the principle that it is only necessary to work an area once in a treatment. In working the pineal and pituitary glands on an infant toe, for example, the adult thumb of the Provider would most often be ringing the bell of most points in the great toe even though the focus or intention is to ring the bell for the specific gland.

Next, stabilize each toe individually as you walk across the tip of each toe to work the skull (#35). The human skull is made up of a number of bones that are joined by soft tissue known as sutures. In babies, the sutures are very soft so that the bones of the skull can mold as the baby's head passes through the birth canal. Later these bones and the sutures become more fixed but do still move slightly. Tension not only affects the neck; it also affects the bones and sutures of the skull. To work the facial bones, do a finger wave with the second and third fingers across the base of the ball of the great toe from the inside of the foot at cervical 1 vertebra (base of the skull) to the inside of the first two toes. This is where the nose and mandible (jaw bone) areas are located on the foot. As you are looking at the bottom of the foot, the vertebrae of the spine and the cranium are in profile with the nose pointing toward the second toe.

To fully affect the eyes, ears, and remaining points associated with the head, do a toe roll for each toe. [*See Figure 3-4*] Stabilize the metatarsal bones, the ball of the foot, with the outside hand while working the toes. Twist each toe gently while rolling between your fingertips from the base of the toe to the tip. Tension in the energy field for the ring muscles of the eyes is also released by this action. People's faces actually change during an SEF treatment because the muscles in the face and head relax.

After working the head area, move to the shoulders (#17). They are located in the fifth zone as discussed previously in the section on the lymph system. Work the whole shoulder area by thumb walking with the outside hand. Do two to three small horizontal stripes from the outside toward the fourth zone. Stabilize with the inside hand. The shoulder energy field can also be worked at the same time as the axillary lymph nodes. After walking the shoulder, bend the toes toward you to view the top of the foot. Your fingers are already in position for doing a finger wave along the base of the toes on the top of the foot. This technique works the collarbone or clavicle (#16).

The thigh (#18) and knee (#19) are located on the outer middle area on the top of the foot. Walk from the top of the thigh to the knee. Pull the toes toward you gently so that you can view the top of the foot. The thigh runs down the side of the instep between the fourth and fifth zones, starting at about the middle of the instep and ending at the knee joint at the beginning of the metatarsal bone. Stabilize the foot with the inside hand and thumb walk down the thigh while stabilizing the fingers of your outside hand on the top of the foot. This hand position takes practice because the thumb is not being walked against resistance from supporting fingers. Your fingers are on the top of the foot so as to ensure that the wrist of your working hand is in correct anatomical position for energy and light to flow through it. The working wrist should never be torqued or turned into a position that causes the elbow and shoulder to rise and torque. Check proper flow position by dropping the shoulder, loosening the elbow, and then placing the wrist and hand on a table with fingertips touching the table. [*See Chapter 1 Figure 1-11*] To work the thigh and knee, the elbow position is rotated only outward so that the thumb can walk the top of the foot toward the toes.

The hip joint is a small point located on the outer area of the anklebone (#20). If the foot is smaller, this point may have already been touched when working the ovaries/testes/base chakra (#9). Use the thumb of the outside hand to ring the bell for the hip. Then place your thumb at the outer edge of the heel and begin walking the large pelvis area in stripes across the heel (#21). I have not found there to be a difference in walking from outer to inner or vice versa, but I remain mindful that there are energy fields for the major blood vessels that flow through the pelvis (depicted on the chart) that may dictate the best practice for working the heel. You can use the thumb-walking technique or knuckles for this large field for the pelvis. The pelvis is a large bone shaped like a butterfly. The lower portion of the wings of the pelvis, or ischium, come together in the midline of the body (and therefore the midline of the heels in SEF) at the pubic symphysis joint. The ligaments of this joint connect the two bones. During pregnancy, for example, these ligaments naturally release so that the woman's pelvis can open more as the baby's head and body are delivered.

RESPIRATORY SYSTEM

From the pelvis area in the heel, bend the toes gently toward you and begin working the respiratory system by walking up the larynx/trachea/bronchus on the top of the foot between the first and second zones. You may prefer to do this in Egyptian hold. The principles to follow for this area of the body are twofold: one, to make sure that your shoulders are dropped in any angle that you take to work the respiratory system so that you can breathe fully and two, to work up this energy field that is the shape of a tube. While the flow of energy is naturally downward toward the lung, many people have allergies and respiratory systems challenged by environmental pollutants that need to be expectorated in the softening mucous produced in the respiratory tract. Working up the bronchus helps the respiratory system to naturally expectorate the mucous. If a person is healthy, there is no harm in directing the movement toward the lungs.

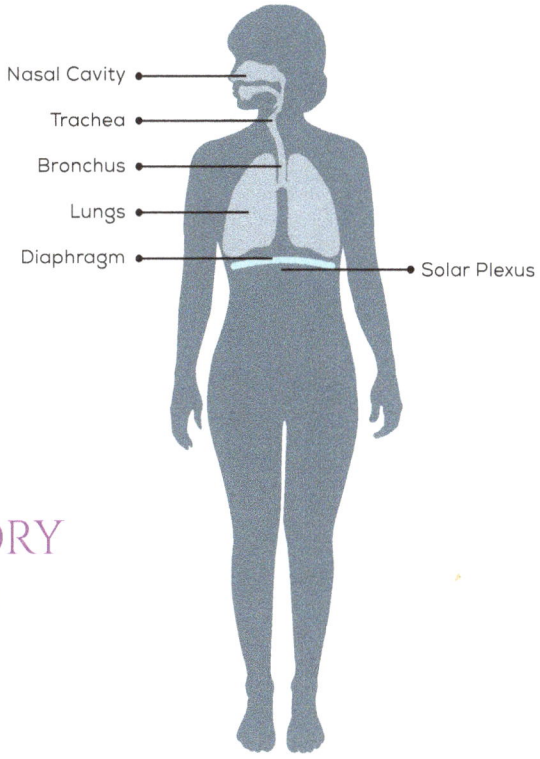

RESPIRATORY SYSTEM

Figure 3-5

Nasal Cavity

Trachea

Bronchus

Lungs

Diaphragm

Solar Plexus

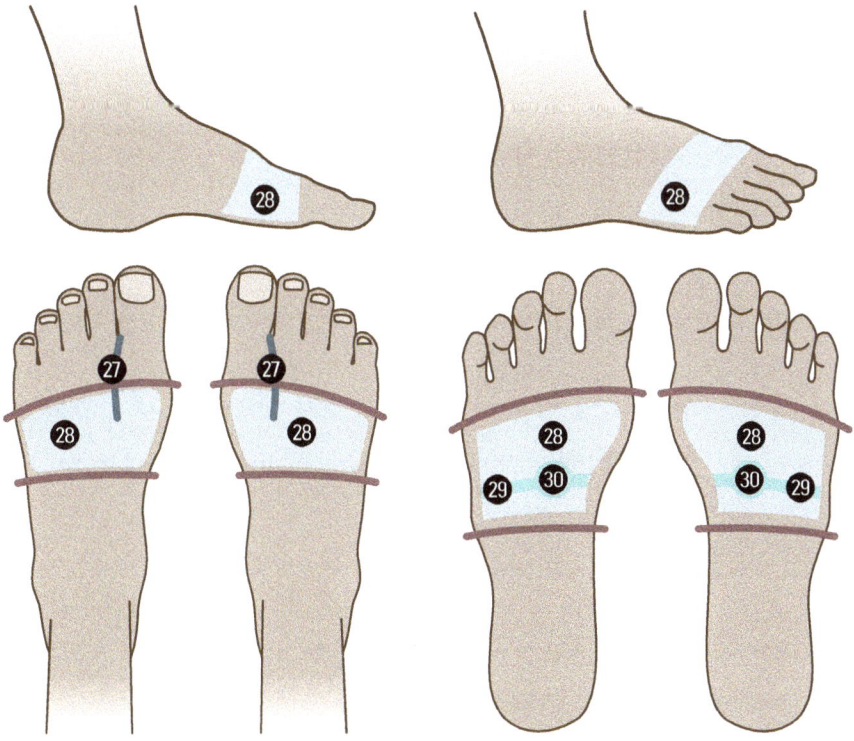

Work the lungs (#28) with the knuckle of the middle finger using a spiraling motion. The lungs' energy field covers the ball of the foot from the second to the fifth zones. After ringing the bell for the lungs over the ball of the foot, place your knuckle into the solar plexus nerve center (#30). Using a gentle spiral motion, work the diaphragm muscle from the solar plexus to the fifth zone and then from the solar plexus to the first zone. The purpose of the action is to release the diaphragm muscle, which is often tight and tense, particularly in adults. Visualize using the spiral action to pull the diaphragm down away from the boney ridge at the base of the ball of the foot. The spiral knuckle action allows for the deeper pulling action on this large muscle where finger walking would only move the energy across the diaphragm. If you find extensive tension in the diaphragm, you can also release it by repeating the solar plexus hold done during the preparation for treatment (See Chapter 1). Releasing the tension in the solar plexus and diaphragm muscle is important because the diaphragm muscle covers all of the zones of the body. Therefore, any tension residing in it affects the organs within all of those zones. The organs of the digestive system are particularly influenced by tension in the solar plexus and diaphragm muscle.

GASTROINTESTINAL SYSTEM

The gastrointestinal system starts with the mouth, where digestion begins. The teeth, tongue, and salivary glands all contribute to the body's ability to masticate and break down food so that it can be metabolized into nourishment for the body. In the hologram of the feet, the mouth (#41) is located under the great toe. The esophagus (#42) is the tube-like organ that follows from the mouth into the stomach (#43). Healthy digestion flows from the mouth toward the

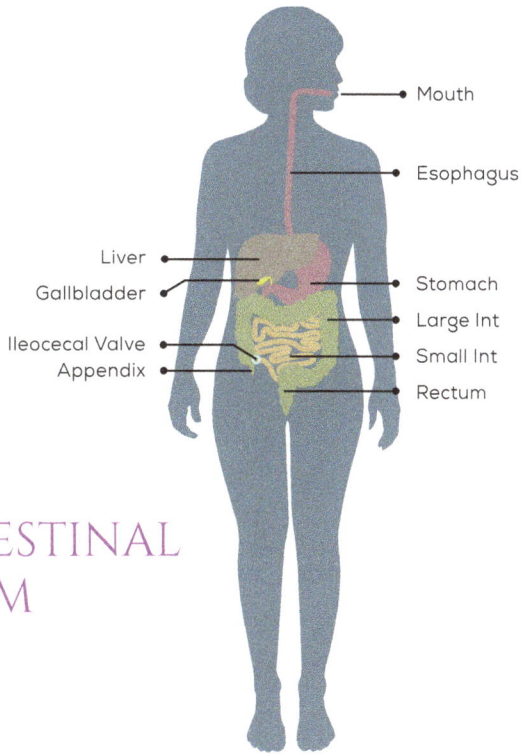

Mouth

Esophagus

Liver

Gallbladder

Stomach

Large Int

Ileocecal Valve

Small Int

Appendix

Rectum

GASTROINTESTINAL SYSTEM

Figure 3-6

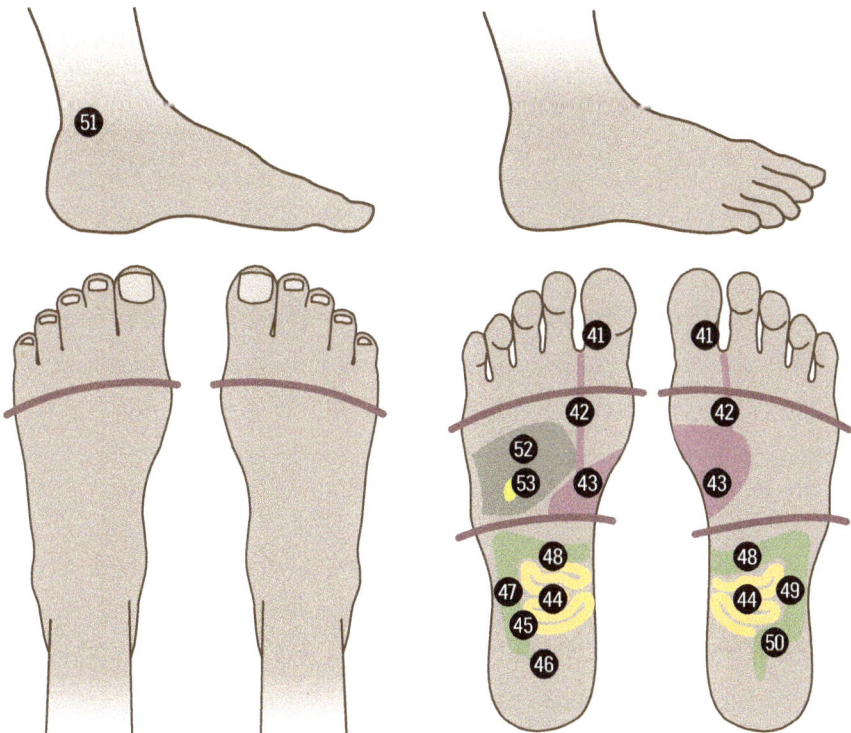

stomach. Follow this flow of energy and thumb walk the pathway from the mouth to the stomach. To send the signal for the mouth (#41) under the ball of the great toe, use either the inside or outside hand. A hook and backup is best used for the mouth point. Continue on, moving to the esophagus (#42). Working the esophagus toward the stomach requires you to lift your elbow so that you can turn your arm and do a forward thumb walk in the direction of the flow of energy through the organs. Do not lift your shoulder or wrist as such lifting creates tension in your hands and can also cause subtle injury over time to the practitioner. This is an important principle to remember in working all points.

Attention to the anatomically correct flow of energy is of particular importance in the gastrointestinal tract because a common malady of people, particularly in industrialized communities, is gastric reflux. Overeating, eating mindlessly, or excessive stimulation of the senses may aggravate reflux. Gastric reflux is one form of "reflux of qi" in Traditional Chinese Medicine, where the energy flows opposite to that which is critical for digestion and absorption of food. The energy refluxes toward the head rather than dropping into the stomach. The valves, which are positioned throughout the digestive system, typically hold back regurgitation of food, but it is the proper flow of energy that provides the direction for this physiological process. SEF treatment of the gastrointestinal system follows the natural flow from organ to organ. In addition, the pituitary gland, which is the master gland that regulates the flow of energy through the valves of the various body systems, has already been treated. Treating the entirety in conditions such as this is described in Chapter 5.

The stomach (#43) is located on both feet. To thumb walk the stomach on the Partner's left foot, walk across the first zone and then into the second zone with your left thumb while supporting the foot with the right hand. To work the portion of the stomach on the right foot, walk across the first zone with your right thumb. After going through the process of digestion in the stomach, food then passes into the small intestine (#44). The small intestine covers four zones. To work the small intestine, use a gentle swirling action with the spiral knuckle action. Visualize moving the food being digested through the tubes of the small intestine and toward the large intestine. The juncture between the small and large intestines is the ileocecal valve (#45), which controls the flow from the last part of the small intestine (the ileum) and the first part of the large intestine (the cecum). This valve can get stuck in an open position as a result of certain foods with tough skins, such as corn and tomatoes. Use a knuckle technique with the middle knuckle of your middle finger to pull the energy from the small intestine toward the lower part of the ascending colon (#47). This technique can help send a signal to close the valve.

The appendix (#46) is a small tail at the very beginning of the ascending colon. Begin the thumb walking of the large intestine at the appendix and move the energy up along the fifth zone of the Partner's right foot. Either hand can be used to walk the ascending colon. Just make sure to move the energy up the fifth zone. However, the left thumb must be used to move the energy across the transverse colon (#48), which begins on the Partner's right foot and continues on the left. Do not thumb walk in the other direction, as this is counter to the natural movement or peristaltic action of the colon's excretory function.

After working the transverse colon on the Partner's right foot, work the liver (#52) and gallbladder (#53). The liver is a large organ located only on the right side of the body. The gallbladder sits up and behind the liver. Its ducts open into the small intestine. Work the liver in three horizontal stripes from the fifth to the second zones.

Walk the thumb with the outside hand underneath the ball of the foot, which is the diaphragm (#29). Walk two more stripes below the diaphragm area. Then using your inside (right) hand, position your middle knuckle on the gallbladder area in the center of the liver field between the third and fourth zones. Push up and in with the corner of the knuckle as if moving behind the liver and rotate your wrist slightly as you then pull and pump the energy of the gallbladder down toward the small intestine area.

When working the Partner's left foot, use your left thumb to continue walking as you move the energy in the transverse colon from the inside of the foot out to the fifth zone where the colon turns downward, known as the descending colon (#49). It can be a bit tricky to work the descending colon. Keeping your shoulder dropped requires that you turn your wrist over and place your fingers lightly on the sole of the foot. Using those fingers for leverage, thumb walk down the fifth zone on the Partner's left foot from below the waistline to just above the heel. At that point, the descending colon enters the sigmoid colon (#50), the S-shaped final part of the colon. The body's fecal matter leaves the sigmoid colon and passes through the rectum (#51) as it leaves the body. The placement of the rectum in the multidimensional hologram of the feet is a challenge. In SEF, it is behind the inner side of the anklebone. Thumb walk up the rectum point with your inside hand. From here, stay on the inside of the foot to work the urinary system.

URINARY SYSTEM

The urinary system includes the kidneys (#37), ureters (#38), bladder (#39), and urethra (#40). This system, like the gastrointestinal system, must be worked in a specific direction following the flow of its physio-

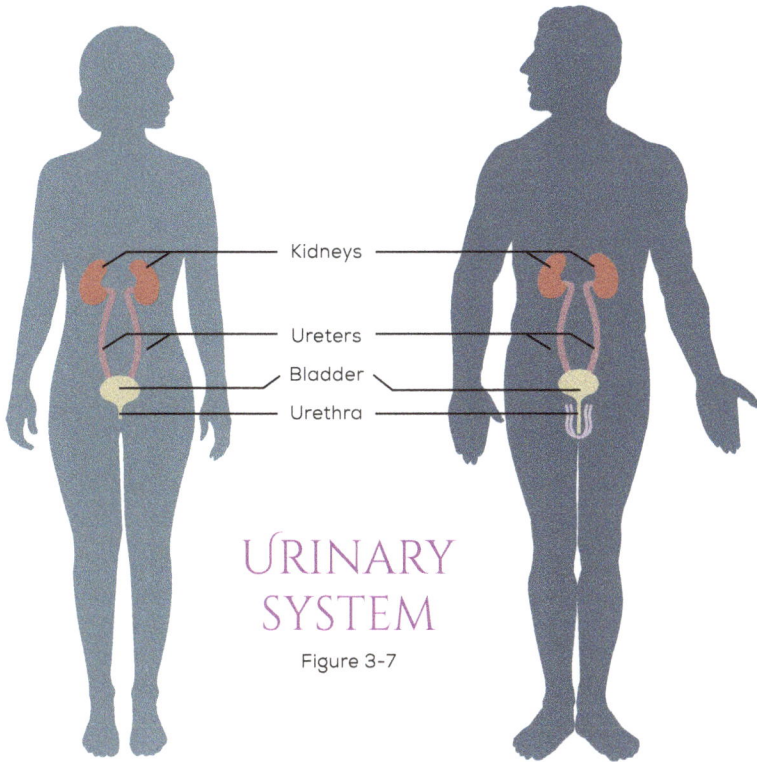

Kidneys

Ureters

Bladder

Urethra

URINARY SYSTEM

Figure 3-7

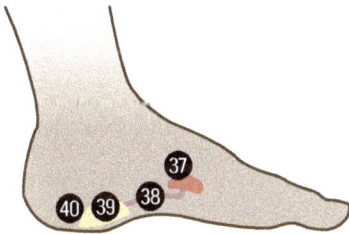 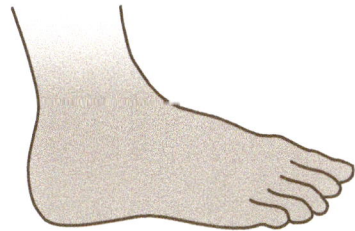

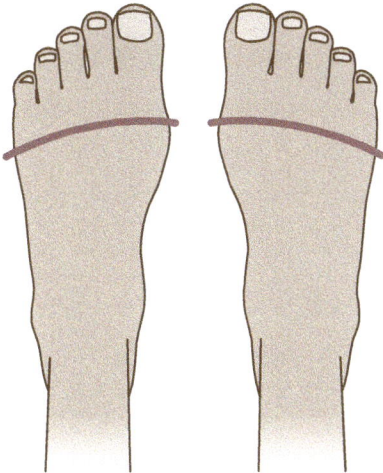 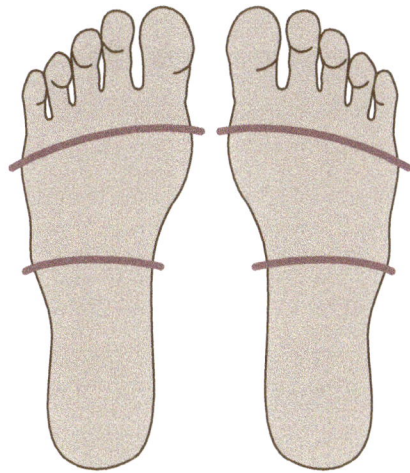

logical excretory function, from the kidneys to the ureters, the bladder and then out of the body via the urethra. Working the opposite direction would move the energy supporting excretion of urine from the body toward the kidneys, an action that would cause severe pathology were it to occur in the physical body rather than energetically. Urine production in the kidneys occurs as a result of the filtration of waste from blood. Blood enters the kidneys through blood vessels going into the center of the bean-shaped organ. It is filtered and then leaves through the vessels. The urine is excreted from the kidneys into the ureters and then held in the bladder until urinated.

SEF hand action models this excretory action. Locate the kidney as done when working the adrenal glands (#5). Working one foot at a time, use a knuckle swirl with your inside hand and support the foot with your outside hand while you move your knuckle over the kidney from the top near the head (toes) to the bottom. Then rotate your knuckle to the center of the kidney and then out toward the ureter. Focus on the excretory flow as you thumb walk the ureter toward the bladder. You can thumb walk the bladder or use a knuckle swirl. The bladder energy field may actually be puffy if a person has to urinate. This is one of the strongest indicators in foot reflexology of the connection between the physical body and the hologram. As discussed previously, the urinary system is located on the inside aspect of the foot rather than the bottom of the foot. Charles always said that if the kidney fields were on the bottom of the feet, they would be stimulated all the time and, consequently, we would be urinating all the time. While the kidney fields are energetically present behind organs on the bottom of the feet, they are more easily accessed on the inner side.

BEING MINDFUL OF THE ENTIRETY
OF THE EXPERIENCE

There are two additional major body systems—the nervous system and the integumentary or skin system—that are part of the SEF experience. However, they are not treated by touching specific points as other organ systems are in the basic treatment. Because they exist throughout the body, the nervous system and skin are for the most part treated in the feet as an entirety. In SEF, the feet and these two systems are affected as an entirety during the general holds and when working the foot through. They are also treated during the herbal applications for stress relief discussed in the next chapter.

Before moving on from the step-by-step system treatment to herbal stress relief, there are some general guidelines for the care of the Partner receiving the basic SEF treatment. First, be mindful that the feet represent the entirety of the body and the person. Mindfulness is a level of consciousness that is expressed in an approach to the healing arts that ultimately manifests as the skill of keen observation. While this book and SEF courses offer guidance in the specific techniques and practices that people have come to know as "SEF," they are not meant to be prescriptive. No education in the healing arts can fully simulate the action that occurs during the healing relationship. Healing is a dynamic process requiring a Provider to be attentive and mindful as to the unique nature of each new experience.

Mindfulness is often first defined as the opposite of mindlessness. Dr. Ellen Langer, a professor of psychology at Harvard University, has defined mindlessness as "automatic behavior," "acting from a single perspective," and "relying on categories or distinctions created in the past to experience our world."[2] Living mindfully means that we

---

2 (Langer, 1989, pp. 10-11)

continually create new categories for registering experience. We are adaptive and responsive without expectations based on past experience and categories.

During a basic SEF treatment, the Partner is re-created as they manifest more and more of their blueprint of wholeness. No two basic SEF treatments given to different people by the same Provider are ever exactly the same. In addition, no two basic SEF treatments given to the same Partner are ever the same. As indigenous peoples say, "We cannot step in the same river twice!" Nature reminds us of the unlimited opportunities in healing. Mindfulness is a state of consciousness that connects us with those very opportunities for healing that are presented to the Provider and Partner alike. A state of mindfulness is foundational to becoming centered in one's whole being. The following is a simple example that Langer cites from Kimble and Perlmutter in her book about how a familiar structure or rhythm can lead to mindlessness:

Q. What do we call the tree that grows from an acorn?

A. Oak.

Q. What do we call a funny story?

A. A joke.

Q. What do we call the sound made by a frog?

A. Croak.

Q. What do we call the white of an egg?

A. Yolk *(sic!)*

Mindfulness is the beginning of preparation to help others. Engaging in the challenge of living mindfully aware of process is foundational for a healthy centering practice (See Chapter 1) that continually clarifies that the focus of healing work is the Partner. Obtain permission from all Partners before conducting the SEF session in which you will intentionally touch their feet. Infants, children, elders, and those who are ill have their own ways of giving consent through body language, verbalizations, and vocalizations. It is a simple thing to do, really. Ask the person, "Would you find it helpful to have an SEF foot treatment?" If the person is not able to speak their consent, watch for physical responses. Obtain consent from family caregivers as well.

It is important to observe your Partner for physical responses at all times during an SEF treatment. Watch their face and body movements and listen to them as they respond to the movement of energy flow. Most of the time, people state that they feel "lighter" and over time their symptom patterns shift in a positive way. There are some responses that, while common, must be addressed during the SEF treatment. For example, a Partner may shiver. This most often happens after the liver has been worked. Make sure that the Partner is covered with a warm blanket; give them a few sips of a warm drink and then hold the right foot with your thumb over the liver energy field. The shivering should abate. Then follow the treatment with the warm castor oil herbal pack described in Chapter 4.

Be very mindful that during an SEF treatment, people may experience pain in various points on their feet as the energy is moved with the action of your fingers and hands. Even a brief ringing of the bell in a certain energy field may be very painful. Assessing the nature of the pain begins with checking your own understanding of anatomy and physiology to make sure that you are as knowledgeable as possible on the subject. Then recheck the landmarks on the foot and make sure that you are sending a signal on the right point/place on the foot. Do not ring the bell for an energy field repeatedly or use brute force. This is unnecessary and unkind. Knowing the amount of pressure to use in SEF to contact a particular point/energy field in the foot is actually quite simple. The force is determined solely according to anatomy and physiology. For example, to reach the gallbladder in the Partner's right foot, you must use a hand action that will go up and under the lower part of the liver energy field. Thumb walking simply moves the energy of the liver, but a spiraling knuckle action can lift the liver (energetically speaking) and contact the gallbladder. The pressure or power of this action is strong but if the gallbladder energy field is flowing well, the Partner will not usually respond in discomfort or pain. *Anatomical contact, not force, is the focus of power in SEF treatment.* Seek correct contact with the various energy fields and let that knowledge be your direction as to how much power enters your hands when you deliver a wholeness current.

There are some important comfort measures you can offer when the Partner experiences excessive pain. Regardless of what point registers a pain response, use a spiraling motion with both hands to work the foot through with the intention of dissipating the energy of the pain response. [*See Chapter 1 Figure 1-17*] This is done calmly and quickly so as not to engage it as you (and your Partner) visualize the energy consumed in the cooling, transmuting violet fire. If the pain has been very strong, you might also choose to do one of the calming holds. [*See Chapter 1 Figure 1-5, 1-6, or 1-8*] The dissipation motion and calming holds in an SEF treatment are the dance between ringing the bell at two points; these in-between point actions are part of the art of the SEF treatment to which you add your own flavor. Just remember to keep moving through the treatment; keep the energy flowing until you have worked the entirety!

Also remember that the signals in babies' and elders' feet are particularly close to the skin surface. Be mindful that your fingers need only provide a lighter touch to contact their signals. Do not breach the pain threshold where a baby screams. While there may be therapies that may advocate for this, SEF does not. My clients have always stated that the pain that they experience is "OK," even "good," in that they say that it dissipates as they feel the powerful release of tension, pressure, stress, stagnation, and discomfort in their bodies as well as their feet during an SEF treatment. By the end of a treatment, they are rested and the stress in their body relieved.

Langer, E. (1989). *Mindfulness*. Reading, Massachusetts: Perseus Books.

◌

CHAPTER FOUR

SEALING OF THE FEET
AND HERBAL STRESS RELIEF

This chapter provides more detail about the herbal stress relief applications used during the SEF treatment—namely the footbath and the anointing with oils. It also addresses the last phase of an SEF treatment, which is the sealing of the feet. The sealing of the feet in SEF is done with herbal wraps and packs. Sealing the feet is an act of protection. During an SEF treatment, people enter a state of relaxation. In this state, they can become open and therefore vulnerable. The SEF Provider protects the person as well as the feet in his/her care by creating a space of kindness, peace, and healing in which the Partner knows they can rest deeply without physical or energetic intrusion of any kind. It is during this time that the Partner can absorb, affirm, and anchor the SEF treatment and any connection with their divine blueprint that has been made.

There are a number of different types of healing spaces and places that can be created in which an SEF treatment can be given. (See Chapter 5) Topical herbal applications are used during the time within the healing space in SEF to create an additional sphere of protection, relaxation, and stress relief. After the basic SEF treatment is completed, an herbal wrap or pack is applied to the Partner's feet and he/she is left to rest with little to no contact for at least five minutes.

During this time, the Partner can process any changes that may have occurred in their body during the SEF treatment. The herbs already introduced to the feet during the footbath and the anointing of the feet with oils are absorbed into the skin of the feet for a deep release of stress and tension and the nourishment of the nervous system.

The nervous system and the integumentary (skin) system were not discussed specifically in Chapter 3. In SEF, because of their anatomical structures and the nature of their physiological functions, these systems—with the exception of the solar plexus nerve center (#30) and the sciatic nerve (#31)—are best treated with actions that affect the entirety or the whole foot/feet. These actions readily occur during the herbal applications. Peripheral nerves are innervated by the central nervous system, which includes the brain and the spinal cord. The nerves are distributed throughout the entirety of the body from the top of the head to the toes and from the inside to the outside of the body. They form a network of electrical signals diffused throughout the skin. The integumentary system of the body defines us in space; with our skeletal system, it is our form. The skin is a boundary that outlines the relationship between our body and the environment. The central and peripheral nervous systems (throughout the skin) are the rheostat or control center where "communications" between our body and the environment are regulated.

While all anatomical systems are part of the whole body, or the entirety, the skin and nervous systems have a particularly integrated relationship with each other and with the chakras. They are connected with the blueprint for the entirety. The nervous system (NS), specifically the sympathetic NS, acts as a transformer for the light energy released by the blueprint and channeled through the heart center and other major chakras. The central NS, which is made up of the brain and spinal cord, comprises the physical components for the communication of impulses throughout the body. This communication is vital instruction for activity that occurs from the organ to the cellular level. When a nerve dies and cells do not get the messages of what to do, they may atrophy and ultimately die.

SEF treatment not only activates organ systems, as the signals for that system are sent from the feet to activate the release of energy from the divine blueprint. It also activates the spaces between systems filled by nerves and skin. While these areas of the body may lack the definition of an organ such as a heart or the liver, these spaces are where energy flow is actually initiated. Just as "dance" is the movement or flow that happens between two actions, it is in these bodily spaces that the activation of flow to and through other body systems begins. Light energy is transformed from the chakras into nerve signals that are channeled through various layers of integument and to the exterior of the body where sensation and interaction with the environment occur.

The five senses, key components of the nervous system, are activated through the treatment of the entirety. The herbal stress relief applications used in SEF bathe, coat, and soothe the skin and peripheral nervous system and, therefore, the entirety. SEF herbal stress relief is helpful in stress management, which is foundational to overall health and well-being. Stress relief is a key to quality of life and longevity. Chinese doctors have for centuries been students of health practices that promote longevity. They sought new practices that would fulfill their commission from their emperor that was to help the ruler outlive the previous one.

What ancient Chinese medicine texts have revealed is that the source of qi in the body is *jing* or essence. Our bodies are endowed at the moment of conception with *prenatal jing*, which supplies the essence for the material formation of our body. Prenatal jing can be likened to an energy bank account and the bank is the kidneys. When the prenatal jing is used up, we die. However, we do not only rely on prenatal jing or essence for our source of energy or qi. Each and every day, we make postnatal jing as well. This jing comes from the food we eat and the air that we breathe. During sleep, any postnatal jing that is not used up for energy is stored as essence. Acquired postnatal essence bolsters the bank account of prenatal jing. The body uses the postnatal jing first, thus allowing the prenatal jing to stay in the kidneys' bank account for as long as possible during a lifetime. As we age, this process becomes more challenged and, ultimately, when we have depleted the postnatal and prenatal jing accounts, we die. Simply put, to live a longer life, plan to make and use postnatal jing and save your prenatal jing for later in life.

Some of the common stressors in life today challenge us and our ability to reserve our prenatal jing. If the food we eat and the air that we breathe are polluted, for example, it is a challenge to create—let alone store—qi that can turn into jing at night during sleep. If we do not sleep deeply, we cannot process qi into jing. From the Chinese point of view, we are only as old as the amount of essence we have consumed—or "we are only as old as our kidneys."[1] Therefore, we must take care of our kidneys. The Chinese philosophy of health and longevity includes the following objectives:

1. Maximizing qi production

2. Minimizing qi consumption

3. Maximizing jing production

4. Minimizing jing consumption

5. Maximizing the health of the kidneys[2]

---

1 (Flaws, 1994, p. 10)
2 (Flaws, 1994, p. 11)

The basic SEF treatment and the herbal stress relief applications help to diminish the negative effects of the stress response by promoting the body's natural responses that can counter such effects. For example, SEF and herbal applications promote deep breathing, deep relaxation, and balance the chakras through the Tau Spiral meditation and signaling of the seven major glands through their counterparts. These seven major glands are activated by stress. The soothing effects of the herbal applications to the nerve endings in the feet and, therefore, the entirety potentiates the possibility of clearing the negative effects of stress that help to manage the kidneys' bank account in addition to the flow of qi. The stress response, which includes the release of the hormone cortisol by the kidneys, is activated by response to environmental stressors. Cortisol release may be helpful initially in those dealing with an immediate danger or those suffering from acute inflammatory response. Over time, if enduring, excess cortisol can increase the vulnerability to infection, memory loss, decreased thyroid function, accumulation of abdominal fat, and increased blood sugar. It is not surprising that foot reflexology treatments are known to be effective in the complementary care of those with health concerns that have a direct link to stress response.

Herbal topical applications used in SEF are powerful but gentle. They soothe the nervous system, which in ancient Vedic texts is likened to a tree called the "triple tree." Yogananda wrote of the origin of the triple tree that, "The two trees of nerves and the life force are condensed out of the tree of human consciousness, the elemental ideas in the causal body, which in turn emanate from Cosmic Consciousness."[3] As we access the triple tree of nerves, consciousness, and life force through the buds of sensation (sight, hearing, smell, taste, and touch),

---

3   (Yogananda, 1995, p. 929)

we contact the elements of Self with a capital "S." This Self is that which is defined in so many healing traditions as being present in nature and all matter as the five elements: ether, fire, air, water, and earth. Throughout the centuries, these five elements have been the framework for the creation of holistic remedies, medicines, therapeutics, and treatments. Holism or whole-ism is represented in treatments or plans of care that integrate the five elements. Herbal applications— footbaths, topical oils, wraps, and packs—provide the Partner with an opportunity for conscious interaction with the elements of Self as the herbs engage the entirety of the hologram that is the whole person— body, mind, emotion, and spirit—through the feet. These simple herbal remedies that incorporate the five elements of nature are applied with compassionate intention. Herbal applications, along with the SEF basic treatment as yogic[4] practice, enable the bond with the Creator and Prakriti[5] to be strengthened and the connection to the divine blueprint opened. Stress relief takes on greater meaning with these holistic herbal applications. Relief is experienced beyond just the physical plane of release of tension in the body. After SEF with herbal applications, the Partner knows the potential for experiencing stress relief as a connection with the Creator through the feet. This is foundational understanding for why herbal applications are important in SEF and why this simple treatment can be so spiritually satisfying and provide opportunity for deep healing.

---

4   Yoga is also defined by Patanjali as "the neutralization of the alternating waves in consciousness . . . then the seer abides in his own nature of self." This refers to his true Self, or soul.(Yogananda, 1995, p. 70)

5   "Mother Nature" the Consort of God...The invisible Holy Ghost creative force. Her production, the human body, is a miniature replica of vast Cosmic Nature. (Yogananda, 1995, p. 891)

FIVE ELEMENT FOOTBATHS

In SEF, footbaths are used at the beginning of the treatment to open the pores and begin the stress relief process. Pores in the integumentary system are openings through which oil is secreted that moistens the skin. The skin is also an excretory organ, meaning that wastes from cellular metabolic processes leave the body through the skin. Just as carbon dioxide gas is excreted through the lungs during expiration and urine leaves the kidneys during urination, metabolic acids leave the skin when the pores open. The skin is often referred to as a "third kidney." Facilitating the excretory function of the skin is something we can do easily with herbal applications to the feet.

The soles of the feet have a high concentration of pores. Helping the pores of the feet to open not only clears waste from the feet but can also support the health of the entire excretory system of the body, including the kidneys where the body's stress is registered. Gravitational pull on the body can promote the accumulation of wastes or metabolic substances such as uric acid in the feet. Reflexologists often feel tiny crystal-like substances come out of the pores of the feet, especially after a hot footbath. I have never had the crystals analyzed but was told by Oma that they were uric acid. Although uric acid is a natural byproduct of healthy metabolism, some refer to the crystals as "toxins." It is possible that over time a buildup of these substances can make the feet toxic or, more specifically, inflamed; so it is best to open the pores and let them be drawn gently out of the feet. The footbaths facilitate this very effectively.

Therapeutic footbaths have been used throughout history in the care and treatment of the ill. They are a part of the therapeutic modality known as hydrotherapy or water treatment. The effects of the bath on circulation, the immune system, and the body as a whole depend upon the duration and temperature of the bath and the herbal remedies integrated with the bath. They are discussed below with suggestions for various applications that can be used in the care and stress relief given to your Partner and the *sealing* of their energy field.

Baths used for sedation need to be at skin temperature of 92°F/33°C. One nursing textbook from the early twentieth century describes the sedative effect of a bath: "A bath at body temperature produces no marked changes in the body, wither thermic or circulatory, but surrounds it with a medium that shields it from all external stimuli, or irritation of nerve endings from air, clothing, pressure, changes in temperature and the like. As a result, the nerve centers and the whole nervous system are protected and allowed to rest. The bath is therefore soothing and quieting in its effects and gives a chance for repair and the storage of vital energy."[6]

The ancient Greeks, such as Aristotle, believed—as did many peoples throughout history—that all matter was composed of the four elements or "archetypes of first matter"[7]: fire was hot and dry; air, moist and hot; water, cold and moist; and earth, cold and dry. These elements and a fifth one they called "pneuma," which referred to vital energy or ether, were considered to be the elements of creation. This early philosophy of healing was applied in Greek medical theory and "humoral medicine" in which the elements were balanced. In contemporary holistic healing, these elements are often referred to as energetic principles. Energetic principles are used when describing people's health patterns as well as in the description of a particular remedy. For example, the main energetic principle of both a person with a fever and the herb Cayenne Pepper is hot and dry. The remedies assigned to this person would be cooling and moistening, such as Peppermint tea. Cayenne (*Capsicum frutescens*) would not

---

6   (Harmer & Henderson, 1939, p. 475)
7   (Hauck, 1999, p. 71)

be appropriate because it is hot and dry and, therefore, would not bring balance to this person's energetic pattern. The environment within and around the person includes the qualities associated with temperature (fire), air (air), fluid (water), and substance (earth). The Hermetic text *The Emerald Tablet* refers to knowledge of the elements of creation as fundamental to the understanding of Self. These Hermetic teachings on Self-knowledge and the elements have inspired many traditions such as Judaism, Christianity, and Islam along with many healers and philosophers from Socrates to Paracelsus to Nightingale. It is the basic premise for the application of herbal remedies in SEF. Knowledge of Self produces awareness, comfort, and peace, all of which are qualities that can ultimately manifest in stress relief. The herbal remedies are used on the feet in SEF in congruence with the ancient wisdom of the five elements and can be a chalice for the manifestation of the alchemy of Self-transformation and promotion of energy flow.

While a footbath is essentially a water element application, any or all of the five elements can be represented in the choices of herbal remedies that are added to the water for an SEF footbath: infusions/decoctions (water), aromatic bath oils (air), bath salt (earth), flowers/leaves (ether), invocation/prayer (fire). The creative choice of herbal remedies used in the footbath is based on your own knowledge of herbs and your assessment of the health patterns you observe in your Partner. For example, if your Partner talks about "having fever for the last week" (fire), you might focus on balancing the five elements by cooling the excess fire with an application from the water element. The water element herbal application for the SEF footbath is the herbal infusion or decoction.

In addition to offering protection, sealing, and balance through the five elements, topical applications like footbaths and anointing the body with oil have been commonly used in the context of relieving fever or inflammation in the external channels of the body.[8] External therapies are adapted energetically to meet the needs of the individual person. There are two types of "fever"—one that is produced of heating factors and the other of cooling factors. The terms "heating" and "cooling" are used energetically and thermally. For example, you can drink a sip of Peppermint (*Mentha piperita*) tea that is warm to the touch (thermal perception of heat), but the Peppermint is actually cooling; it cools the heat in the head. Cooling herbs and essential oils from cooling plants are used to cool the "fever" caused by heating factors. Warming herbs and essential oils from warming plants are used to warm a "fever" due to cooling factors. This way of using herbal applications to create a balanced environment for healing is powerful in its simplicity. A translation of this ancient teaching means that a careful assessment of the Partner as a whole person (entirety) in terms of their thermal qualities is the foundation for the choice of herbal applications in SEF. Thermal quality is ranked on a scale: cold – cool –neutral –warm – hot. See the following chart of SEF topical herbal applications for examples of cooling, neutral, and warming SEF herbal topical applications. The use of a thermal scale is a beginning approach to the application of essential oils in SEF. While an SEF practitioner may go on for further education in the use of herbs and their constituents, such as essential oils as is done in aromatherapy, the knowledge of topical herbal applications provided in this book is sufficient for application in a basic SEF treatment to offer significant stress relief.

---

8   (Dash, 1988, pp. 165-166,Vol. 3)

THERMAL QUALITY	COOLING	NEUTRAL	WARMING
Massage Oil **E = Essential Oil** **I = Infused Oil**	Mint (E); Eucalyptus (E); Grapefruit (E); Lemon (E); Lemongrass (E); Melissa (E); Wintergreen (E)	Rose (E); Geranium (E); Lavender (E); Calendula (I); St. John's Wort (I)	Sesame (I); Chamomile (E); Sandalwood (E); Ginger (E); Rosemary (E); Myrrh (E); Castor (I)
Poultice/Plaster **(Whole Herb)**	Cucumber; Aloe	Hops	
Compress **(Cloth Soaked in Herbal Infusion/ Decoction)**	Witch Hazel Distillate; Lemon; Digestive Bitters; Tea	Calendula	Swedish Bitters; Ginger
Footbath	Mint; Melissa; Lemon; Orange Blossom; Lemongrass; Eucalyptus	Lavender; Hops; Rose	Thyme; Rosemary; Chamomile; Valerian

Each of the following five sections highlights a topical application commonly used in SEF to seal the energy field of the feet. Each of the five herbal footbath applications represents one of the five elements of Self: water, earth, fire, ether, and air. The Partner can be offered a choice of these footbaths for stress relief. People often choose the application and element that suit them best. Health practitioners who have knowledge of how the five elements work with healing traditions, such as Traditional Chinese Medicine, Ayurveda, or holistic nursing, might include additional insight for their clients' choices according to those traditions.

Infusions and Decoctions in a Footbath for the Feet (Water Element)

The SEF footbath was described earlier in the book. This section focuses on the herbs that may be chosen to create the sealing, protecting, and stress-relieving effects. Many plants can be extracted in water and added to a footbath to induce one of these effects. The medicinal qualities of plants are extracted in water by two methods: infusion and decoction. Both are commonly referred to as "tea." The difference between infusion and decoction is the way in which water is used. In the infusion process, gentler parts of plants such as leaves and flowers are immersed in boiled water for 5 to 15 minutes. In decoction, the harder part of plants, such as roots, stems, barks, berries, or seeds, are boiled for 15 minutes up to 1 to 2 hours. The harder dried herbs are always steeped in water that has been raised to the boil for 4 to 8 hours before decoction to allow for the plant material to soften and expand for easier extraction into the water. Leaves and flowers do not need to be pre-soaked.

Supplies for an Herbal Infusion or Decoction:

- Fresh or dried herb: 5 to 10 grams of leaf or flower heads or up to 30 grams of dry root per liter or quart of water
- Cutting board and knife
- Water (distilled or spring)
- Sauce pan – stainless steel
- Cheesecloth or fine sieve

Method:

1. Must be done ahead. Prepare an herb infusion/decoction to be poured into the bath water.
6. Fill the footbath basin with warm tap water.
7. Using cheesecloth or sieve, strain the infusion/decoction into a separate bowl, glass jar, or pitcher. Secure the opening of the cheesecloth and press remaining liquid from plant material.
8. Pour infusion into basin.
9. Check the water temperature for comfort.
10. Allow the Partner to soak their feet for 20 minutes; this is the amount of time the pores take to open fully. This ideal amount of time may not be feasible in some settings and situations. Adapt as needed. You may also choose to place a blanket over the Partner's shoulders during the footbath if they feel cold.

Examples of Herbal Infusions and Decoctions for a Footbath:

The best and ultimately safest way of partnering with any plant in creating a remedy such as a footbath is to first be introduced to the plant. Get to know the plant. Plants are amazing teachers that will tell you everything you need to know. Here are some suggestions for where to start:

Thyme *(Thymus vulgaris)* warms the chest. It has significant antimicrobial and antiviral properties, making it a good option during cold and flu season, particularly for seniors. Thyme's aroma may be less familiar than lavender or rose. It is a common culinary herb and one of its constituents is the leading ingredient in the original version of the antiseptic mouthwash Listerine. Have your Partner sniff it first. If your Partner likes the smell, remind them to breathe in the aroma during the footbath.

Coffee *(Coffea arabica)* warms the abdomen and the energy channels in the body. It can also act as a stimulant for the liver and large intestine. The Coffee footbath is an old nurses' remedy for headache that is used to draw the energy from a person's head toward their feet. Many Coffee drinkers may not think of their daily bean beverage as an herbal decoction, but it is.

Chamomile *(Matricaria recutita)*: Its name originated from the Greek chamos (ground) and melos (apple), alluding to its growing low on the ground and to the apple-like scent of its fresh flowers. The therapeutic uses of Chamomile flowers are recorded in the works of ancient physicians Hippocrates, Galen, and Asclepius. Egyptian tradition consecrates Chamomile as a sacred herb of the sun and, therefore, an excellent remedy for fever. An infusion of the flowers (no leaves or stems) is anti-inflammatory inside and out. Have your Partner sip a little Chamomile tea if they choose this plant as their footbath. Chamomile also relieves sinus pain and stuffiness.

Mustard *(Brassica nigra or alba)* is best known for its ability to increase the sensation of heat in the body and to relieve pain and congestion. Topical applications of Mustard have been used historically for sciatica, gout, and other joint pains. Mustard increases circulation at the surface of the body. This process of stimulating the skin is known as counterirritation. The oil of the Mustard seed is a very strong irritant. Take care. If it is applied to the skin in its pure state, it will cause immediate blistering; but, if properly prepared and diluted, it can reduce pain in the joints of the feet. Hot water poured over black Mustard seeds can also help with pain and discomfort related to colds and headaches.[9] Some pharmacies still sell dried Mustard bath preparations that can be added to footbath water.

Aromatic Bath Oils (Air Element)

Many of the herbal preparations used in footbaths during SEF treatments are chosen for their aromatic properties. While herbal infusions and decoctions can be more accessible in that the herbs are often found in the kitchen or garden, concentrated herbal bath oil preparations are very convenient in that no cooking is required. Smaller volumes are used because they are concentrated, thus making them more portable and easy to store for immediate use.

Have your Partner choose their bath oil. You might have them sniff two or three choices and pick the one they like most. Watch your Partner's face for positive reaction. There are many brands of herbal bath oils on the market. Make sure when you buy them to purchase only those made with *medicinal grade* pure essential oils extracted from plants as opposed to manufactured fragrance oils. Fragrance oils are those found in potpourri, for example.

Oma introduced me to Olbas® bath oil in the 1980s and I have offered it ever since. It is a Swiss formula, which includes a proprietary blend of essential oils of Peppermint, Eucalyptus, Cajuput,

---

9   (Grieve, 1971)

Wintergreen, Juniper, and Clove in carrier oil. It also includes chlorophyll, which gives it a deep green color and makes it cooling to sore and tired feet. Following Oma's tradition, I also offer other European brands of bath oils, such as Kneipp and Dr. Hauschka/WALA. Plain essential oils such as Rose, Eucalyptus, and Rosemary can be used in a footbath (5 drops per liter or quart of water); because essential oils are used in SEF after the footbath, it is rare to use straight essential oils during the footbath.

Examples of Aromatic Herbal Bath Oils for a Footbath:

Thyme and Chamomile (See Infusions and Decoctions section)

Rosemary *(Rosmarinus Officinalis)* has a long history of traditional use for increasing circulation and warmth as well as for relieving joint pain and stimulating the mind. Rosemary leaf's antioxidants and other compounds may work to prevent oxidation and the breakdown of acetylcholine in the brain, leading to a potential prevention and/or suppression of the symptoms related to dementias. The Camphor in Rosemary leaf is a known stimulant for the central nervous system, respiratory system, and circulation. Elderly patients often experience a warm Rosemary footbath as the best remedy for helping to ease the discomfort related to the generalized aches and pains and cold extremities they experience, especially when they are in an unfamiliar place such as a hospital or nursing home.

Lavender *(Lavendula officinalis)* has been used for centuries in countries such as India for psychiatric disorders. Lavender essential oil has the ability to bring balance to body, mind, and spirit in that it both relaxes and stimulates. Lavender is used specifically for depressive states associated with chronic digestive disturbances. It is used as an antispasmodic, sedative, antidepressant, and antirheumatic as well as to relieve fatigue and expel intestinal gas. Lavender oil is used topically to increase circulation and regenerate cells of the skin. In Ayurvedic medicine, Lavender is called the "broom of the brain" because its use is said to sweep away sluggishness of thought, strengthen brainpower, and clarify the intellect. The essential oil is also used to ease colic and chest congestion, and to relieve biliary complaints and headaches. Warm moist applications of the flowers help relieve pain associated with rheumatism and neuralgia. Lavender essential oil is especially analgesic.

Melissa/Lemon Balm *(Melissa officinalis)*: The word "balm" is an abbreviation of "balsam," which means fragrant oil. The leaf has a light lemon and mint fragrance. The ancient Greek and Roman physicians used Lemon Balm leaf steeped in wine for both internal and external maladies. It has been used topically for surgical wounds and to treat venomous bites and stings. Old European texts record the use of Lemon Balm to improve memory. In Anthroposophical practice, Lemon Balm infusion or oil is used to bring about an "airing through" of the whole organism to balance the relationship between water and air. Conditions associated with insufficient "airing through" are intestinal and menstrual disturbances, and nervous disorders.[10] Psychologist Carl Jung prescribed Melissa baths for melancholy (sadness) and to strengthen the memory. The leaf is also a common remedy to induce sweating and to alleviate fever during colds and flu.

Hops *(Humulus lupulus)*: The traditional uses of Hops include applications to improve the appetite and promote sleep. Hops are used for their relaxing, diuretic, and pain-relieving properties. They are given in cases of nervousness and hysteria as well as to induce sleep in instances of extreme agitation. Hops are also used in heart disease, nervous disorders, and neuralgia. They are used as a digestive tonic in jaundice, indigestion, liver complaints, and bladder irritation.

---

10   (Husemann & Wolff, 1982)

Hops are said to be effective for delirium tremens, a condition related to the withdrawal from excessive and chronic use of alcohol. Certain plant therapies are often used in the spring to support the liver's natural tendency to become more active after the winter. Traditionally, a small glass of Hops tea is taken three times a day in the spring to stimulate a "sluggish liver." An old recipe for a syrup made of the juice of the plant and sugar was known to cure jaundice, ease headache, and cool sensations of heat in the stomach.[11]

Bath Salts (Earth Element)

Bath salt is important to consider when your Partner says that he or she has very tired or sore feet, very tense muscles, or calloused and dry feet. Salt softens the hard water that most often comes out of the tap. The skin of the feet can be softened significantly with a salt bath. My friends and aromatherapists Kathy Keville and Mindy Green use this recipe for Aromatic Bath Salts:[12]

Supplies:
- 1 cup borax
- ½ cup sea salt
- ½ cup baking soda
- 50 drops essential oil (1/2 teaspoon)

Method:

Mix the dry ingredients together and add the essential oils, mixing well to combine. Use ¼ to ½ cup bath salts per bath. For a footbath, use approximately ¼ cup of bath salts per tub. For muscular

---

11   (Culpeper, 1990, Originally published in 1814)
12   (Keville & Green, 2009, p. 88)

aches and pains, the addition of ½ cup Epsom salts to the basic recipe can be very helpful. Epsom salts are also the preferred salt for those who feel energetically depleted or vulnerable. For example, women going through menopause and soldiers in the military often benefit from the anchoring action of the earth element by the addition of bath salts to the footbath.

Floating Flowers and Leaves (Ether Element)

Ether is the vital energy essential to the other four elements. The ether element can be integrated into the SEF footbath through the addition of selected flowers and leaves. Flowers and leaves are simply floated on the surface of the water in the footbath. The radiation of their beauty and fragrance (if any) can be absorbed through the pores and the energy field of the feet. This is a very subtle energy healing technique that is well known in the beauty and resort industries. Rose petals floated on the bath water, for example, emit a very subtle fragrance as well as fill the bath water with essential oil molecules that have gentle relaxing and even hypnotic effects. The healing power of plants is extended much beyond their molecules and biochemical effects. Dr. Edward Bach of England, who founded the self-care system called *Bach Flower Essences*, spoke in 1931 in Southport, England, of the healing power of beauty in nature in his address *Ye Suffer from Yourselves:*

> *Those beautiful remedies, which have been divinely enriched with healing powers, will be administered, to open up those channels for the reception of our Spiritual Self, to flood our natures with the particular virtue we need, and wash out from us the fault, which is causing harm. They are able, like beautiful music, or any gloriously uplifting thing, which gives us inspiration, to raise our very natures, and bring us nearer to our Souls; and by that very act, to bring us peace, and relive*

our sufferings. They cure, not by attacking disease, but by flooding our bodies with the beautiful vibrations of our Higher Nature, in the presence of which disease melts as snow in the sunshine.[13]

Any of the "38 Healers"—the Bach Flower Essences healing system—can be used in the bath as well. These essences come in little bottles and are sold as a set or individually. To help your Partner choose a flower essence to use in the bath, you would match what they say about their state of mind or mood (the pattern) with the Flower Essence as it is described in terms of the mental and emotional conditions it affects and the "positive potential" that can emerge in the person "once harmony is restored" after using the remedy.[14]

Actually, any plant and its essence can be invited to the footbath. I often create a special bath with plants much the way I make a flower arrangement for someone. The only difference is that I use only a small representative of the flower or plant, such as a single bud, leaf, or flower head. Prior to harvesting the flower or leaf from the garden, I place some tobacco or a copper penny at the base of the plant as an offering in exchange for the medicine I am bringing to the client. Over the years, I have seen the most powerful healing in my patients who have harvested their own herbs and flowers in my garden. Participation in choosing, harvesting, and making medicine as in the herbal footbath provides direct access to the gentle healer within the Partner. If you have a garden, you might consider offering your Partner the opportunity to harvest their flower or leaves for their footbath before you begin the treatment.

---

13   (Bach, Howard, & Ramsell, 1990, p. 62)

14   (Howard, 1996) Instructions on the use of this self-care system of 38 Flower Essences and Rescue Remedy formula are also found on the Bach Centre website: http://www.bachcentre.com/centre/select.htm

Invocation and Prayer (Fire Element)

The fire element is exemplified in warmth and heat. While the footbath is often warm, it can also be cool. A cool footbath is particularly refreshing for feet during the warm summer months when people's feet swell more easily from walking on the pavement or ground warmed by the sun. The fire element is also represented in the warmth of the heart and the passion of the voice (throat chakra) asking the Creator for the Partner's healing.

Before starting the SEF treatment, you would have meditated and centered, allowing you to focus your energy in the heart. Invocation and prayer are expressive creative acts in which the fire of the heart is raised to the throat chakra and the power released in sound. Invocation and prayer are part of ancient healing practices. Many cultures' healing traditions are passed from generation to generation through spoken or sung verse rather than written. Within many of these ancient traditions is the acknowledgement of the source of healing, the Creator. The Creator conveys healing through the descent of *light*. Light from the Creator is the origin or source of energy flow. This is why the invocation "Let there be Light!" is a simple invocation used in SEF. Using your heart and throat or power chakra, call the light of the Creator into the water and herbs in the footbath. Bathe the feet in light and the fire of your heart! Activate the fire of the heart with feelings of love, care, and understanding.

INFUSED AND ESSENTIAL OILS

Herbal oils (also called oil infusions to distinguish them from essential oils) are made by saturating fresh or dry plant material with a fixed oil such as olive or safflower oil. The oil is massaged into the skin for various reasons, depending on the plant used. For example, the flowers of **Arnica montana** are infused in oil and can be rubbed into sprains and sore muscles. St. John's Wort oil (*Hypericum perforatum*) can be applied for nerve pain.

Supplies:

- Use fresh or dried plant material, depending on which plants are best used as oils and whether they must be prepared from fresh or dried herbs. You may need to do some research to answer these questions. Some plants, such as St. John's Wort, must be used fresh.
- Widemouthed glass jar with cheesecloth
- Rubber band to use as cover
- Oil

Method:

An oil of the flowers and tiny leaves of the St. John's Wort (SJW) plant are used as an example here. SJW oil is applied to first- and second-degree burns and is used in wound healing and for muscle and trigger point pain, particularly nerve pain. The aerial parts of the *fresh* plant (flowers and small leaves) are collected, chopped, and placed in a widemouthed jar. A little oil is added to the plant material and then the flowers are crushed again with the back of a spoon. Then more oil is added to cover the plant material completely. The jar is shaken and placed in a warm location for 10 days to two weeks. The oil must be approximately 38°C or 100°F during the infusion time. SJW oil turns red in color due to a constituent in the petals of the flower.

After the oil infusion has turned red, the plant material is strained out of the oil. The residual oil is then pressed out of the plant material with cheesecloth. Because fresh material is used, some water may still be in the herbal oil even though the cheesecloth covering allows for some evaporation. The water can cause the oil to go rancid over time, so it is best to let the strained oil sit for one week undisturbed. The oil will rise above any water remaining and can be decanted off into brown glass storage bottles.

If dried plant material is used to make an herbal oil (herbs other than SJW), grind the dried herb to a powder when you are ready to make the oil. Wet the herb thoroughly with oil and stir. Add oil so that the level is a few centimeters above the herb powder. Cap the jar tightly and put in a warm place. The same method is then followed as with fresh herbs like St. John's Wort, except that dried herbs absorb the oil. The oil level must be checked after the first 24 hours, and more oil is added if needed.

Liniments are lighter topical remedies than oils and are usually alcohol or Camphor based for quick absorption by the skin. Liniments have been used traditionally to warm and stimulate muscles and ligaments. They evaporate quickly so that no oil is left on the skin as with herbal oils. Liniments are often used before physical exercise to warm up the body, but they can also be used for local inflammation after exertion. Liniments are used in specific areas of the body rather than for full-body massage. The herbs traditionally used as liniments are the more warming herbs like Cayenne and Lobelia. One of my favorite liniments is a Camphor-based liniment with Lobelia that is applied to the temples for discomfort related to headache, migraine, and eyestrain. The Camphor, as with all alcohol-based liniments, is cooling, while the herb is warming. Liniments feel initially cool on the skin and then quickly begin to warm.

Aromatic essential oils are used in making the massage oils used in SEF anointing. Essential oils are extracted from aromatic plants. They make up a very small amount of the whole plant. Essential oils evaporate readily and, therefore, once extracted, must be kept in sealed bottles. They are sold in small amounts because they are a highly concentrated plant constituent. For medicinal purposes, they must be used in pure form. Aromatic oils often are considered precious and valuable and are used in small amounts. Like perfume, essential oils are used in small amounts that do not overpower the sense of smell. Some essential oils are lighter in fragrance than others. For example, Lemon Verbena is less intense than Cinnamon.

The Partner should always give input into the choice of the aromatic oil used on their feet. Make it part of your practice to have the Partner sniff anything you plan to put on their feet the first time. Essential oils also can be blended for specific medicinal effects related to the absorption of the properties of the oil through the skin and the inhalation of the scent. Aromatherapy, like homeopathy, is a healing art related to herbal medicine, but because it is a specific science and art in its own right, it is studied as a separate subject. SEF is not aromatherapy; essential oils are simply applied in the anointing of the feet and "working through" the feet.

Essential oils from aromatic plants affect the health of body, mind, and spirit. Throughout history, perfumers have known of the medicinal benefits of the aromatic volatile oils they used. Religious rituals continue to include the aromatic use of plants as incense, such as Frankincense (*Boswellia carterii*). The olfactory cells are the only place in the human body where the central nervous system comes in direct contact with the external environment. Humans' sense of smell is one direct connection with their environment. Plants often provide that sensory experience. The essential oils from plants have specific healing properties such as relaxation effects, antimicrobial properties, and the ability to raise mood and spirit.

Blending Herbal Massage Oil

Herbal oils, used for anointing and massage, are made with drops of essential oils in a light carrier oil, such as Sweet Almond oil, which has no fragrance. Aromatherapists Keville and Green suggest that the most therapeutic action of essential oils occurs when the scent is "very faint, just barely detectable."[15]

Supplies:

- Carrier oil (Sweet Almond oil)
- Essential oils (medicinal grade)
- 1-ounce glass bottles with glass dropper

Method:

To prepare a 2% to 3% dilution, use 10–12 drops per 1 ounce/30 ml of carrier oil. This can be used for healthy adults. Prepare a 1% dilution using 5 drops per 1 ounce/30 ml oil for pregnant women, people with illness, and children. In SEF, do not make blends with Eucalyptus or Pine essential oils. Eucalyptus is used in the ablution and Pine oil on the feet can cause a burning sensation if it were to come in contact with heat during the Castor oil foot pack that is applied at the end of the treatment.

Choose only high-quality essential oils. Get to know the properties and qualities of every oil that you decide to use. Keep it simple and study well before applying the essential oil with your Partner. Start with four or five essential oils, such as Rosemary, Lavender, Rose, and Lemon. Essential oils considered "base notes" as in perfuming are heavier and longer lasting in a blend. These oils, such as Myrrh, Jasmine, Frankincense, Rose Absolute, and Sandalwood, linger after the oils considered "top" and "middle notes" in a blend evaporate.

---

15   (Keville & Green, 2009)

Top notes include Eucalyptus, Grapefruit, Lemon, Lemongrass, and Peppermint and middle notes include Chamomile, Geranium, Clary Sage, Fennel, Lavender, Rosemary, and Thyme.

Blends include representatives from the three categories of notes in varying proportions. When blending, first place a drop of the oil on a paper towel or strips of blotter paper until you find a fragrance that you find satisfying. Do not test on your skin as the fragrance of the oils changes when they come in contact with skin. Reserve a 1-ounce bottle for a specific Partner in your personal apothecary. You might also consider designing a "basic" massage oil blend to which you can add a drop of a middle or base note given your Partner's preference. The following are four examples of basic topical massage oil blends I have used that have allowed me to easily personalize the oil for each Partner/patient at the time of treatment. I pour about a teaspoon of the base oil in my hand and add one drop of the base note chosen by the Partner. After coating my hands with the final oil, I have the Partner sniff it before applying. Do not rub the oil into your own hands as the purpose is to anoint the Partner's feet without excessive interference from your own body oil or energy. Once you establish that a basic blend works well for your Partner, you can blend these basic massage oils in a larger 4-ounce/120 ml bottle. Proportions may need to be adjusted based on the quality and source of the essential oil.

2. Pain Relief (Neutral to Cooling) For External Use
   a. 6 ml/120 drops Lavender essence
   b. 3 ml/60 drops Wintergreen essential oil

3. Uplifting (Cooling) For External Use
   a. 2 ml/40 drops Lemongrass
   b. 1 ml/20 drops Rose
   c. 1 ml/20 drops Sandalwood

4. Soothing (Neutral) For External Use
   a. 2 ml/40 drops Lemon
   b. .5 ml/10 drops Wintergreen
   c. .5 ml/10 drops Fennel

4. Stimulating (Warming) For External Use
   a. 4 ml/80 drops Rosemary
   b. .5 ml/10 drops Ginger

WRAPS AND PACKS

Wraps and packs are a lost art and science in contemporary medicine and nursing, but they are preserved in allied health sciences of physical and occupational therapies and in the spa, massage, and body workers industries. In SEF, the herbal wraps and packs are applied to nourish the skin of the feet, open and draw out uric acid from the pores of the feet, and seal the energy field of the feet. The two most common wraps/packs used in sealing the feet following the basic SEF treatment are the Castor oil and Swedish bitters packs.

The use of oils coats and soothes the nerve endings in the feet. This is best accomplished by a wrap or pack that is snug to the foot and ankle and secure during movement. I often think of the pack experience as a mother offering security to her child by tucking them in at night. The feet represent the whole person and their soul (sole). The delicacy with which we care for the soul can be expressed in the detailed attention to the security and comfort of the soul during the herbal pack. Principles of applying a pack to any part of the body include:

1. Move as quickly and smoothly as possible when applying the pack so that the feet do not get chilled.

2. Each layer of the pack is secured within the next layer of material so as to seal in the herbal oil and keep out air that will cool down the pack (in the case of a hot moist pack).

3. Assess frequently for comfort. Pull the fabric during application so that bunching and wrinkling do not occur. This is particularly important if a person is going to walk on their pack for any length of time.

Castor Oil Pack

I first learned the benefits of a warm, soothing Castor (*Racinus communis*) oil pack or compress from a healer who had been affiliated with the Edgar Cayce Foundation in Virginia Beach, Virginia. Edgar Cayce (1877-1945) was a medical clairvoyant for 43 years whose work included numerous plant remedies. Cayce recommended Castor oil packs in cases of impaired lymph flow; inflammation; congestion; constipation; gallbladder, liver, kidney, and pelvic disorders; muscle spasms; and back pain.[16] Castor oil is very viscous compared with other oils and when placed on the skin provides a protective coating that penetrates the tissues very deeply. With the assistance of heat, the oil is taken up readily by the skin and tissues to provide a calming effect. Oma translated the Castor oil pack to the feet. She referred to the Castor oil pack as "dessert" because it is applied after the "main course," the basic treatment.

Supplies: [*See Figure 4-1*]
*   Cotton flannel cloth (two swatches 14 in x 14 in)
*   Castor oil
*   2 plastic bags (large, plain – made for loaves of bread)

---

16 (Duggan & Duggan, 1989)

- Two (thin, not plush) hand towels and one large bath towel
- Hot-water bottle filled and burped (optional)

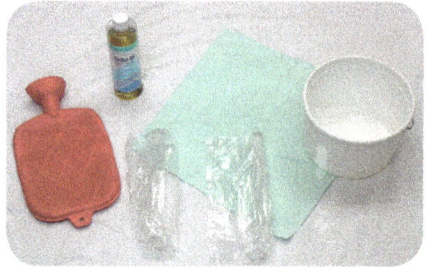

4-1   CASTOR OIL PACK SUPPLIES

Method – Castor Oil Pack to the Feet:

There are two ways of preparing a Castor oil pack for the feet or any part of the body. The Cayce method is to completely soak a wool flannel with warmed Castor oil and apply it. In SEF practice, I use another method

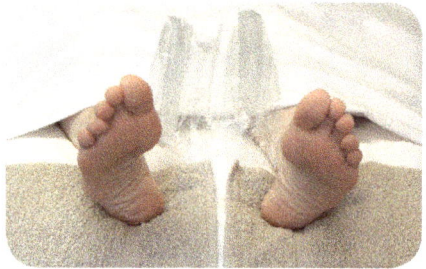

4-2   PREPARATION

with warm moist heat that requires significantly less oil because the oil is applied directly to the feet. Before coating the feet with oil, open the plastic bags and gather them so that they can be put on to the feet quickly. Place them near the feet. [*See Figure 4-2*] The feet will already be positioned on the towels. The large towel is placed under the feet after the footbath and the two hand-size towels are placed one under each foot after the footbath to be used to cover the foot when it is not being worked. Lay the towel horizontally under the foot with the heel of the foot about 2 inches from the inner side of the towel. [*See Figure 4-3*] The long end of the towel on the outside of each foot that looks like a flag can then be

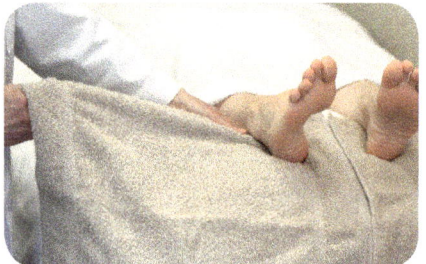

4-3   TOWEL PLACEMENT

grabbed easily to use as a cover for the foot when needed.

Once the feet, plastic bags, and towels are in position, pour up to 1 tablespoon of Castor oil into your hand. The amount needed will be determined by the size of the feet, but you should use enough oil to thoroughly coat the feet so that they are shiny all over. [*See Figure 4-4*] The hand motion is to coat the feet. Do not rub the oil into the skin. Do not wipe the oil off your hands because the oil will provide protection to your hands during the next part of the application in which you will use very hot water! Using a small bowl or bucket, wet the flannels in water that is steaming and as hot as you can manage. Wring out the flannel so that it is not dripping. Hold the square-shaped piece of flannel in front of you and rotate it with the point turned upward like a diamond. Place the top of the diamond

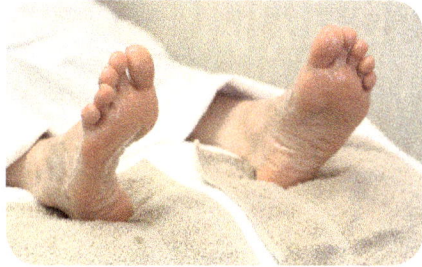
4-4   CASTOR OIL ON FEET

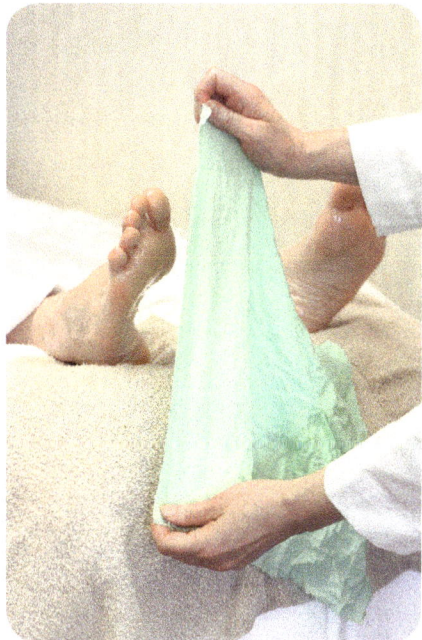
4-5   POSITIONING THE FLANNEL

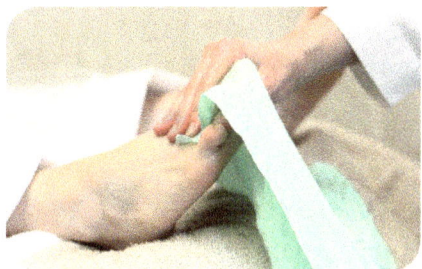
4-6   WRAPPING THE FLANNEL

over the toes; wrap each side around the foot; then bring the back point up around the heel. [*See Figures 4-5 through 4-9*] Work quickly so that the flannel remains steamy. Turn the scrunched bag so that one of the corners is by the toes and the seam of the bottom of the bag along the sole of the foot. Draw the bag over the foot and up the ankle and gently push out the air. [*See Figures 4-10 and 4-11*] Secure it with one hand as you begin to wrap with the towels.

Each small hand towel is wrapped around the foot. Wrap the corner of the hand towel nearest you over the toes; wrap the inside 2 inches of the towel and secure it with your inside hand. Use your outside hand to turn the edge of the towel nearest you over slightly; stretch the towel out away from the foot to create a light tension in the towel and then pull back over the top of the foot and then around it. The towel fits

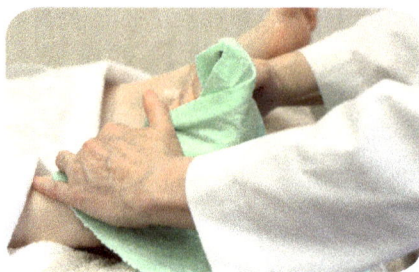
4-7 WRAPPING THE FLANNEL

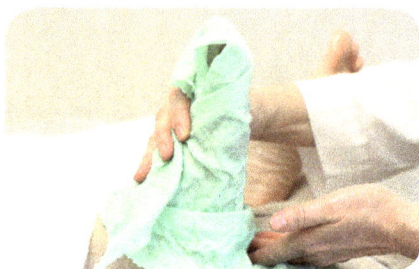
4-8 WRAPPING THE FLANNEL

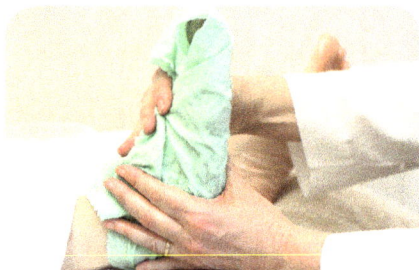
4-9 SECURING THE FLANNEL

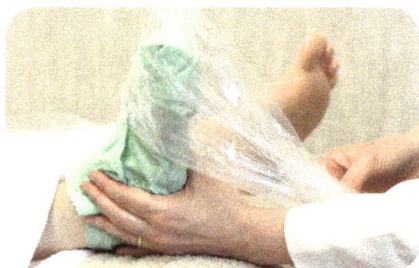
4-10 COVERING WITH BAGGIE

snugly around the foot and a corner tucked in by the ankle. [*See Figures 4-12 through 4-18*] After both feet are wrapped and tucked in, they are placed side by side at the center of the bottom edge of the larger towel. At this point, you can opt to place a hot-water bottle at the bottom of the feet outside the small towels if you are planning to leave the pack on for a longer time. The hot-water bottle helps to keep the pack warm. Then fold the edge of the large towel nearest you up and over the pack (and bottle). Wrap the inside of the large towel around the feet, securing the bottle in place. Wrap the other side of the large towel around the feet and secure. [*See Figures 4-19 through 4-24*] Each layer of the pack should cover the previous layer so that air does not enter the pack. Cover the feet with the sheet that is over the patient and then with a warm blanket. [*See Figures 4-25 through 4-27*]

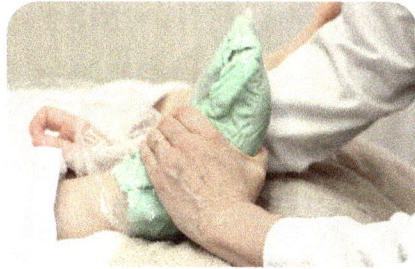

4-11   PUSHING THE AIR OUT

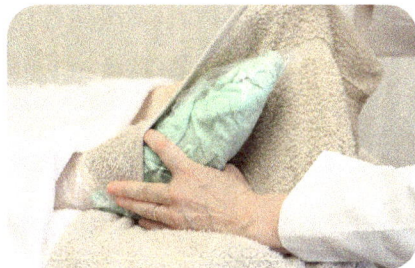

4-12   WRAPPING THE HAND TOWEL

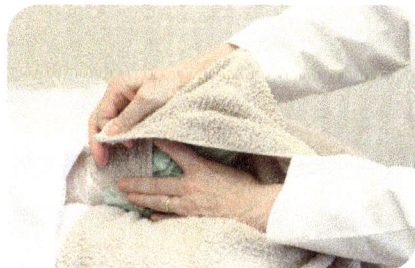

4-13   WRAPPING THE HAND TOWEL

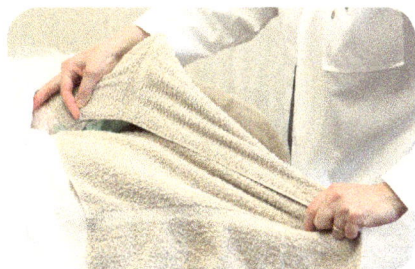

4-14   STRETCHING THE HAND TOWEL

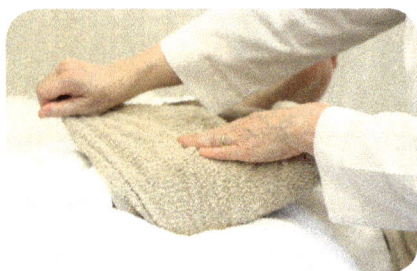

4-15   WRAPPING THE HAND TOWEL

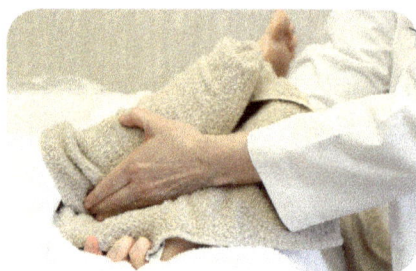

4-16   WRAPPING THE HAND TOWEL

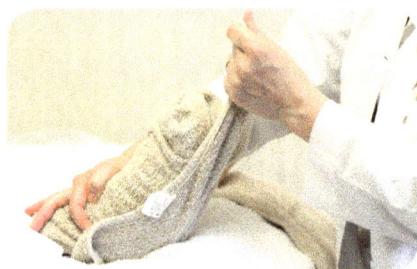

4-17   SECURING THE HAND TOWEL

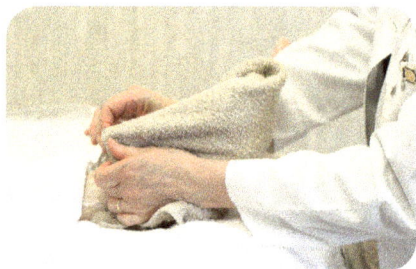

4-18   SECURING THE HAND TOWEL

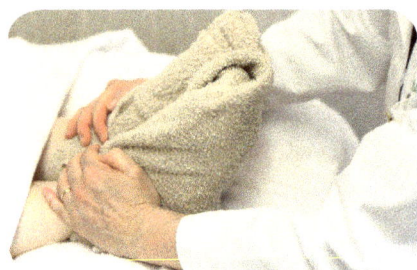

4-19   PUTTING THE FEET TOGETHER

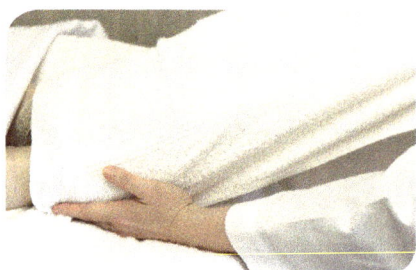

4-20   WRAPPING THE LARGE TOWEL

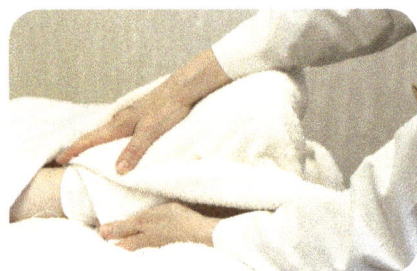

4-21   WRAPPING THE LARGE TOWEL

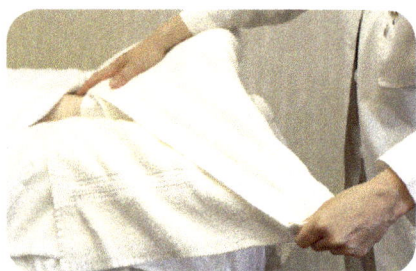

4-22   STRETCHING THE LARGE TOWEL

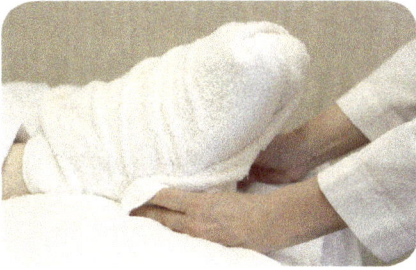

4-23   SECURING THE LARGE TOWEL

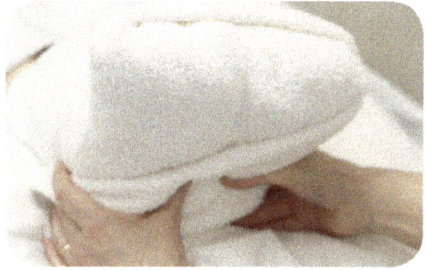

4-24   SECURING THE LARGE TOWEL

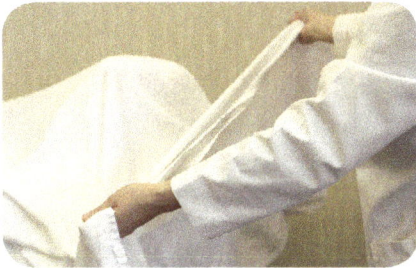

4-25   COVERING WITH THE SHEET

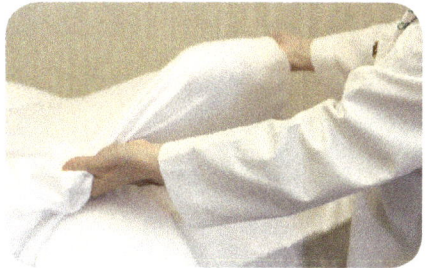

4-26   SECURING THE SHEET

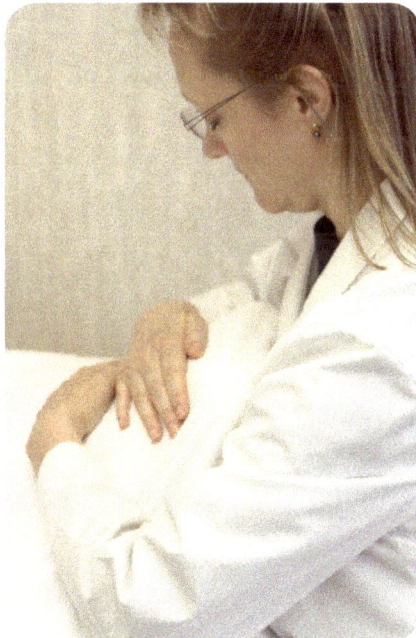

4-27   PROTECTING THE SOLE WITH YOUR HEART

Leave the Castor oil pack in place for 5 minutes up to 1 hour depending on your time frame for the SEF treatment. Dry packs (without moist heat and hot-water bottles) can be left on for hours. If the moist pack is very hot, the oil will be readily absorbed. Be sure to look closely at the feet when you take the pack off to see if the oil was absorbed. If not, you did not make a pack that was hot enough. Go back through the steps and practice. It takes awhile to learn the skill and art of applying Castor oil packs to the feet. Remove the pack quickly and open the towels one foot at a time. Draw the flannel into the plastic bag with your fingertips by scooping the pack and bag down the ankle and foot. Try not to touch the flannel. Keep the flannel in the plastic bag until it is washed or discarded. After the pack is removed, cover the foot immediately with the hand towel to keep the foot warm. Wipe between the toes if there is any residual oil. See below for the finishing treatment.

Swedish Bitters Pack

One of Oma's favorite herbal remedies was bitters. Medicinal plant bitters, a combination of bitter plants, are used in European herbalism as well as Ayurveda and other healing traditions to aid digestion. In Ayurveda, bitter taste is known to restore the sense of taste. A common bitter plant used in bitters is Dandelion leaf (*Taraxicum officinalis*). My mother used to harvest Dandelion flower heads in the spring to make a vat of Dandelion wine that was drunk at dinner to aid digestion.

Bitters are made from herbs that are extracted in alcohol rather than water as in an infusion or decoction. Oma's preferred recipe for bitters was "Swedish Bitters," a recipe found among the writings of Swedish physician Dr. Claus Samst and made popular by the renowned German healer Maria Treben. The Swedish Bitters remedy is discussed in the book she published in German and English, *Health Through God's Pharmacy*.[17] The herbs in the formula include Myrrh, Saffron, Senna leaf, Camphor, and Rhubarb root. In the spring, (in the Northern hemisphere) when temperatures begin to get warmer, the liver energy starts to move more after being dormant during the cold winter months. Bitter herbs and bitters help to move the energy of the liver. Traditionally, bitters are taken internally; a small amount of extract is put in warm water or herb tea. In SEF, Swedish bitters may be applied to the soles of the feet. This is called a Swedish Bitters Pack.

Some packs can be soothing and drawing like the Castor oil pack while others are more stimulating. The bitters pack is stimulating, particularly for the digestive system and the liver. This pack can be part of an annual health ritual of "spring cleaning" for the liver or it can be applied in the care of those who are healing their livers, such as after taking certain medications like antibiotics or pain pills. The pack is typically put on the feet after the footbath and the oils used on the feet have been absorbed during the SEF basic treatment. A Swedish

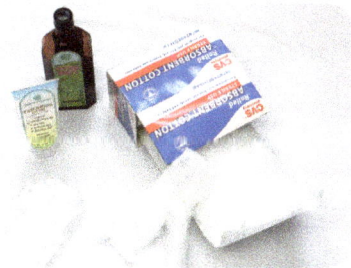

4-28   SWEDISH BITTERS PACK SUPPLIES

Bitters Pack is used in lieu of a Castor oil pack.

Supplies: [*See Figure 4-28*]

- Swedish Bitters Liquid Alcohol Extract (approximately 1 ounce per foot)
- Calendula cream
- Rolled cotton cut to length of foot (measure from base of toes to start of heel)

---

17   (Treben, 1999)

- Plastic sheet or bags cut to the size of sole of foot

- Cotton or silk socks (have Partner bring clean pair of socks). To prepare the sock for application to the pack on the foot, scrunch it and push the toe to the opposite side. Set it down near the Partner. [See Figure 4-29]

Method:

1. Rub a small amount of Calendula cream into the soles of the feet. This will nourish the skin of the feet and also protect the skin from irritation or itching from the bitters.

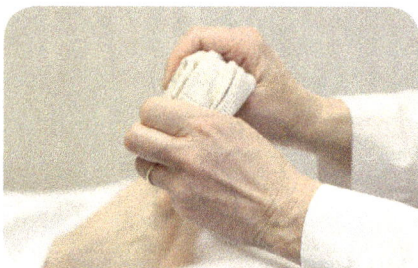

4-29 PREPARE THE SOCK

2. Take the rolled cotton cut to size and open it into two halves. [See Figure 4-30] Mold one piece into a ball and slowly dribble the Swedish bitters onto the ball as you squish the cotton to promote absorption of the bitters. [See Figure 4-31] The goal is to use as little bitters as possible so that when applied to the feet, the bitters will not leak but stay absorbed in the cotton.

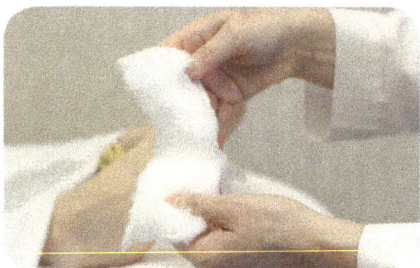

4-30 CUT AND OPEN THE COTTON

3. When the cotton is coated and brown, unfurl it and

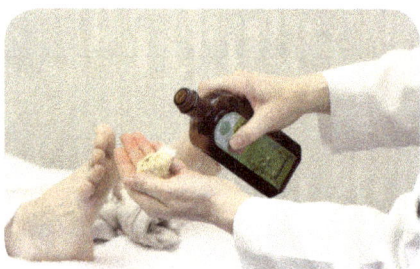

4-31 SATURATE WITH SWEDISH BITTERS

mold it onto the sole of one foot. Place the thin piece of plastic under the foot and hold it with one hand over the toes to secure it while you put the sock on the foot. [*See Figures 4-32 through 4-34*]

4. Put the scrunched sock over the toes first; grab hold of the toes and secure the sock and pack in your hand. Use the other hand to unfurl the sock over the pack. [*See Figures 4-35 through 4-37*] Your Partner can then walk in their shoes or sandals with the pack secure.

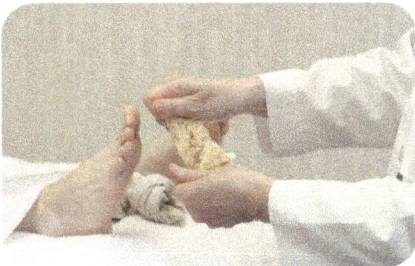

4-32   UNFURL THE COTTON

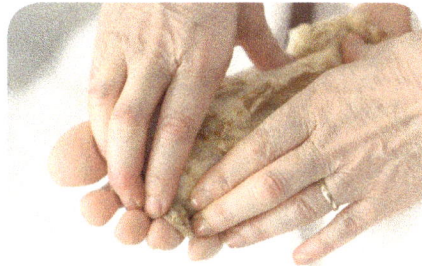

4-33   MOLD THE COTTON

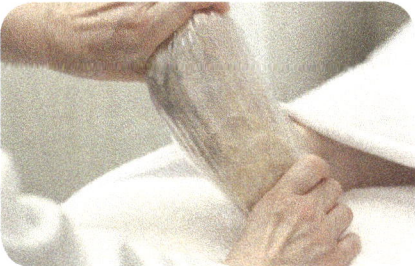

4-34   PLACE THE PLASTIC

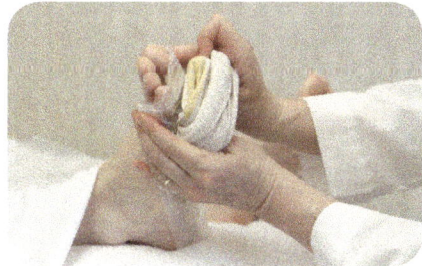

4-35   PLACE THE SOCK

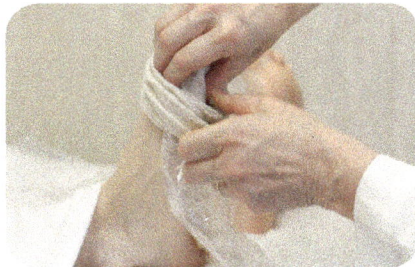

4-36   GRAB THE TOES AND PACK

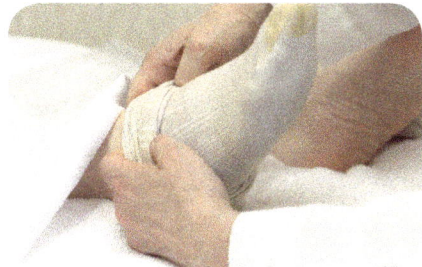

4-37   UNFURL THE SOCK

ADDITIONAL NOTES ON SEALING THE FEET AND HERBAL STRESS RELIEF

Some herbal infusions or decoctions can be given as tea to sip throughout the SEF treatment to facilitate energy flow within the body, connection with the blueprint, and stress relief. Consider the following herbal beverage teas:

Mint *(Mentha spp.)* assists in cooling and clearing the head and sinuses. Use 1 tsp. of the dry or 2 tsp. fresh leaf infused in 1 cup boiled water.

Cinnamon *(Cinnamomum verum)* assists in opening and warming all energy channels in the entirety. Use 3 small to medium sticks for 2 cups of water. Lightly boil for 30 minutes.

Nettles *(Urtica doica)* assist with adjustment to life changes and transitions and reactivity to the environment, such as allergy and hyperactive airway/asthma and skin irritations. Use 1 tsp. dried herb infused in 1 cup boiled water.

Coffee *(Coffea arabica)* assists with headache and low mood. Aids stimulation of the liver and large intestine. Brew the coffee for the optimum time of the grind of bean you select (fine, medium, coarse, etc.).

Horsetail *(Equisetum arvense)* assists with rehabilitation from bone fractures and structural change. Use 1 tsp. dried herb infused in 1 cup boiled water.

Eleuthero *(Eleutherococcus senticosus)* assists in adaptation response to excessive stress. Supports adrenal glands. Use 30 drops of liquid alcohol free extract in a small amount of boiled water.

Lemongrass *(Cymbopogon spp.)* assists in raising mood and spirit. Use 1 tsp. dried herb infused in 1 cup boiled water. Serve with relaxing, nourishing oatmeal cookies.

Elderberry *(Sambucus nigra)* assists in opening the pores during a cold and the flu. Use 1-2 tbsp. of the syrup in warm water.

There are some finishing touches that are applied after the pack. Be sure to look at the feet after the pack for any redness of the skin. As you work the feet through using a spiral motion with both hands, ask your Partner how his or her feet feel. Most people report that their feet are "lighter!" Place one drop of Peppermint massage oil (blended as described above for a 1-ounce bottle) on your fingertip and run your fingertip along the spine from the sacrum to the base of the skull under the big toe. Walk the spine one more time, visualizing the light rising up the spine.

Oma based her instruction about using the Peppermint along the spine on a spiritual teaching on healing that she had heard. After applying this technique for two decades, I decided to look more deeply into the healing tradition and traced it to my own spiritual roots in Agni Yoga. I have been a student of the Agni Yoga teachings of Helena and Nicholas Roerich since the 1980s. A museum featuring their work is located in New York City[18] where I had been working as a professional dancer and choreographer. Nicholas's paintings have been the inspiration for some of my dances. Mdm. Roerich's writings on life, spirituality, and healing are profound. She recommends rubbing Mint leaves along the spine for relief of the pain in the spine due to the awakening of the Kundalini.[19] Rubbing Mint (Mentha spp.) along the spine can also be used for dispelling imperil. Mdm. Roerich defined imperil as "the poison resulting from irritability that attracts danger" and is "deposited against the walls of the nerve channels and then spreads throughout the organism."[20] These deposits of imperil are painful and contribute to the decomposition of matter, including

---

18   See www.roerich.org and www.agniyoga.org . For a brief history of the Russian Philosopher Helena Roerich, see http://en.icr.su/family/hir/index.php

19   (Roerich, 1929, pp. 140 - 141 #220)

20   (Roerich, 1929, pp. 15-15 #15)

the body. Mdm. Roerich wrote, "If modern science would try to examine objectively the nerve channels, giving heed to the astral currents, it would encounter a strange decomposition of the astral substance during the passage of that substance through the nerve channels—this is a reaction to imperil."[21] This imperil is very stressful to carry physically, emotionally, and spiritually.

Mdm. Roerich wrote of Mint, "One should remember that during the departure of the astral body the physical remains unprotected, and if the air is poisoned, the appearance of undesirable guests is unavoidable. Mint is the best disinfectant. It also aids the astral body, which leaves the physical body more often than we think."[22] Fresh Peppermint leaves can be used in lieu of the Mint massage oil. Pluck a few leaves from the stems and rub them gently along the spine on each foot from base (#11) to neck (#14).

SEF treatments simultaneously open the channels to the descent of light from the Divine blueprint of wholeness while clearing the feet and energy field of imperil and the stress it imposes. So many people identify with the negative energy in their energy field even when it is not their own. The feet walk the earth and readily pick up on the energies positive and negative. SEF treatments provide the space and time for the reflection on these energies stored in the body and the nerve endings, and to practice discernment in ridding the body of imperil through such practices as the Mint leaf ablution.

After this final ablution and sealing, work the feet through one last time with the intention of "closing the door" to the feet. Hold the feet and speak an invocation for the sealing and protection of the healing energy released during the SEF treatment. It is not

---

21   Ibid.
22   (Roerich, 1929, p. 126 #196)

a requirement of the SEF treatment, but do consider ending with a simple act of love and compassion that the Partner can carry with them when they leave. I like to put the Partner's socks on for them before they get up and then bring their shoes to them. Kindness is demonstrated in simple acts. All herbal remedies are applied with kindness toward the Partner and to the plants for the offering they have made to human healing. Kindness is the remedies of remedies.

Bach, E., Howard, J., & Ramsell, J. (1990). *The Original Writings of Edward Bach*. Essex, England: C. W. Daniel Co.

Culpeper, N. (1990, Originally published in 1814). *Culpeper's Complete Herbal and English Physician Enlarged*. Glenwood, Illinois: Meyerbooks.

Dash, R. K. S. B. (1988). *Caraka Samhita*. Varanasi: Chowkhamba Sanskrit Series Office.

Duggan, J., & Duggan, S. (1989). *Edgar Cayce's Massage, Hydrotherapy, and Healing Oils*. Virginia Beach, Virginia: Inner Vision Publishing Company.

Flaws, B. (1994). *Imperial Secrets of Health and Longevity*. Boulder, Colorado: Blue Poppy Press.

Grieve, M. (1971). *A Modern Herbal*. New York: Dover Publications.

Harmer, B., & Henderson, V. (1939). *Textbook of the Principles and Practice of Nursing* (4th ed.). New York: The Macmillan Company.

Hauck, D. (1999). *The Emerald Tablet*. New York: Penguin Group.

Howard, J. (1996). *Bach Flower Essences for the Family: An Introduction to the Basic Principles and Standards of the Bach Flower Essences and a Guide to Their Use*. London: Wigmore Publications, Ltd.

Husemann, F., & Wolff, O. (1982). *The Anthroposophical Approach to Medicine*. New York: The Anthroposophic Press.

Keville, K., & Green, M. (2009). *Aromatherapy : A Complete Guide to the Healing Art* (2nd ed.). Berkeley, California.: Crossing Press.

Roerich, H. (1929). *Agni Yoga*. New York: Agni Yoga Society.

Treben, M. (1999). *Health through God's Pharmacy*. Steyr, Austria: Ennsthaler Verlag.

Yogananda, P. (1995). *The Bhagavad Gita*. Los Angeles: Self-Realization Fellowship.

CHAPTER FIVE

✧

CONCLUSION: THE FLOW OF HEALTH PROMOTION AND HEALTH CARE REFORM

The flow of kindness—from the heart, head, and hands—to the Partner is the channel through which all healing intention must pass. It carries a certain vibration that is felt by the hearts of others. Kindness is universal consciousness. It is the source of unity and peace, personal and planetary. Teachings on kindness are found in many cultures. Yogananda taught kindness as the foundation for spiritual life. He wrote that the practice of being kind as practice of the yogic ideal includes: "wearing the fine garment of genuine courteous language," remaining calm in disagreements, being charitable (that is being concerned for the feelings of another), viewing all people as brothers and sisters, and demonstrating "affection for all of God's creation."[1]

Kindness is our natural state and yet there are so many obstacles that seem to challenge and impede its expression every day. SEF provides the opportunity for the creation of daily spiritual practice, that is ritual, that actively draws down waves of light that empower the expression of kindness in healing service to humanity, heart,

---

1   http://www.anandaclaritymagazine.com/2014/03/kindness-foundation-spiritual-life/

head, and hand. SEF is an antidote to unkindness in all forms. SEF activates energy flow and dispels the physical, mental, emotional, and spiritual manifestation of imperil that gathers on nerve endings as crystallized irritability, a seed that can spawn unkindness. One of the mantras I like to repeat as I am creating an SEF treatment with a person is one that I learned from the writings of Mdm. Roerich on flow. She wrote that, "He who is afflicted with 'imperil' must repeat, 'How beautiful everything is!' And he will be right; because the flow of evolution is rational, in other words, beautiful. The more subtle the nervous system, the more painful is the precipitation of 'imperil.' This same poison, by the addition of one ingredient, may contribute to the dissolution of matter."[2] SEF, created within a healing environment of kindness and beauty, can offer an opportunity for healing and peace to a person, but that act has an effect on all life. Just as the drop of a single pebble causes the flow of water to ripple outward, touching all parts of a pond, so too can the wave of kindness and beauty from an SEF treatment ripple outward, leading to healing and peace for all. This is the beauty of the potential of SEF. It is also the awareness of this potential that causes one to pause and realize the importance of understanding that, with the potential, comes responsibility for ensuring the safety of the practice.

SAFETY AND SUPPORT GUIDELINES

There are some basic safety and support guidelines that are foundational for an SEF treatment. These guidelines for practicing SEF attend to the physical, mental, emotional, and spiritual needs of the Partner and Provider. Many of these have been mentioned already, but are highlighted here to emphasize their importance.

---

2   (Roerich, 1929, p. 16)

1. **Sleep and Rest:** Sleep is critical in dealing effectively with the imperil and planetary effluvia that the feet come in contact with on a daily basis. When you offer an SEF treatment to someone, you also engage with his or her imperil and contact with planetary effluvia. Therefore, it becomes imperative to give the body adequate time to rest and sleep. Giving a treatment is typically very energizing for the Provider because the practice of connecting with the divine blueprint can dispel your own blockages in energy flow; nevertheless, the body must have sleep. You must be able to discern which physical symptoms in your own body mean that you must rest before treating another. If you treat when your "battery" is low and/or your ability to connect is challenged due to any life stressor, the fountain of energy you need to be will not be present and there is a risk that the treatment will not move or clear the Partner's energy at all. A treatment given without permission of the body can easily become an energy drain for a Partner. Sometimes, all that is needed is a 10-to 15-minute nap to tap into the "Source." Short naps, under 20 minutes, have been shown in studies to be very effective in recharging the energy in the body in contrast with longer naps. During sleep, the dream state can serve as a place for inspiration and inner guidance for SEF healing work.

2. **Entirety:** An SEF treatment attends to the entirety. The underlying philosophy of SEF is that the whole body and its systems are related. Therefore, an SEF Provider would not treat a separate part. For example, a person might say that they have a headache. Although the Provider would benefit from this information and take note of it, he or she

would still give the whole SEF treatment with the focus on the entirety of the feet and not simply on the head area. If someone were constipated, an SEF Provider would not offer to work the large intestine alone. This is an important distinction between the dominant biomedical system in which a person and their health concern is often reduced to a focus on a particular part of the body or the mind. This reductionism also lends itself to biomedical diagnosis and treatment, which is not the purview of SEF. SEF is about energy flow and, therefore, the entirety—the whole sphere of influence that is both feet—must be addressed in a given SEF session.

3. **Hand Washing:** Hand washing is an effective way to prevent infection and strip effluvia from your energy field. Wash your hands before and after each client. Rinse your forearms with cold water from the elbows, allowing the water to run from the elbows to the hands and off your fingertips. You will know that you have taken on the effluvia from your Partner's feet when your hands or forearms feel heavy. The cold-water ablution relieves the heaviness. You may also experience pain, particularly shooting pain in your thumb, hand, wrist, or forearm as you work on the feet. Be sure that you are centered and that you rinse with cold water as soon as you can, such as during the pause between the treatment and before applying the pack.

4. **Feet Inspection and Consent:** Before and after the footbath, inspect the feet. Carefully note any open sores, bruises, cuts, and structural deformities. Be sure to mention any of your findings to the Partner. The Partner may dismiss

the findings as insignificant, but that is your consent to help them. You should, however, not touch damaged skin. Use only a light touch over deformities until you get to know a person's feet well. Your notation serves as a record of any physical concerns with the feet prior to SEF. Do not treat without consent and affirmation that the Partner actually wants to have an SEF treatment. At Golden Apple Healing Arts, people can buy gift certificates for SEF. When someone calls for an appointment, it is important to give a brief explanation of what SEF is and then ask if they are interested. While an SEF treatment with a consenting adult might be informational for them, healing can only really occur when an adult affirms the possibility for their healing.

5. **Footbath:** Only touch the water to test the temperature and diffuse the chosen herbal remedy into the bath water. Use a two-step disinfection process to clean the basin after a footbath. Scrub the foot basin with hot, soapy water and rinse. Then spray or rinse the basin with a cold or room-temperature 10% bleach solution and allow it to dry.

6. **Use of Essential Oils:** Never use essential oils undiluted and do not use them internally. Use only medicinal-grade essential oils. Keep all oils out of the reach of children.

7. **Stop:** Know when to stop. Be quite mindful that you accurately locate the energy field for the area of the body you intend to work on. Follow the SEF instructions—"ring the bell," visualize, and send a signal. Other foot reflexology schools of thought give different types of instructions for how to gauge the amount of pressure to use. In SEF, the instruction as outlined in this book is quite specific:

Learn anatomy and physiology, use the landmarks for the feet as shown in the SEF chart to accurately locate a field on the unique Partner's feet, ring the bell, and visualize as instructed. In addition, tickling is a sign of stress. Oma called ticklishness in the feet "synthetic stress." She remedied the ticklishness by treating the feet even when the person laughingly mouthed the word "stop." She would always stop briefly to check in and the client would urge her to continue. I find that the ticklishness often resolves during the footbath if the Provider is very focused and purposeful in their touch.

8. **Dragging the Skin:** Dragging the skin creates an unnecessary pain response. Always move forward when you are thumb walking so as not to drag the skin on the feet and create a burning sensation. Use spiral motions when working the feet so as to avoid dragging the skin.

9. **Uric Acid:** Uric acid is thought to be the cause of blockages on the nerve endings of the feet. These blockages are then reflexed to the corresponding organs and systems of the body. One of the aims of foot reflexology and Foot Zone Therapy is to rid the feet of these uric acid blockages. Therefore, it is not in the best interest of treatment for the Partner to consume foods that potentially contribute to the buildup of uric acid in the body. These foods include those high in purines that lead to the development of uric acid, such as organ meats, herring, anchovies, alcohol (red wine), high-fructose corn syrup, mushrooms, spinach, asparagus, and cauliflower. My Foot Zone Therapy teacher, Charles, also told his clients that they could not eat citrus fruits. He had been made aware of some studies in Russia in Olympic athletes whose kidney function diminished significantly when eating citrus.

10. **Explanations:** Choose your words carefully and do not over-reach in conveying what is known about the understanding of the science underlying SEF. Be sure to stick to conveying to your Partners what the experience of an SEF treatment can be like. For example, when explaining a pain response in the feet, you might say, "That is blocked energy in the large intestine area of the hologram in the feet" rather than "That is your large intestine," which can suggest a problem with the actual organ. Identifying problems is not the purpose of SEF. Moving energy is.

11. **Pregnancy:** Foot reflexology can be used by a knowledge-able practitioner to facilitate labor. Therefore, unless you have been trained by a knowledgeable practitioner, do not give a full SEF treatment to a pregnant woman. You can, however, offer them a soothing footbath. Do not use very hot water or perform the ablution with its downward strip-ping action. Hold the feet instead, allowing for the woman to commune with her unborn baby while relaxing in the footbath. During summer months, cool footbaths can be very helpful to women whose feet and ankles have become swollen. Do not use essential oils or strong bath oils blended from essential oils when caring for pregnant women.

12. **Precautions:** If someone is on pain medication, realize that their pain response, a protective mechanism that is gauged in the SEF treatment, has been altered and may affect their response during an SEF treatment. You may not be able to treat this person without risk.

13. **Frequency:** The frequency of foot treatments varies but is generally provided on a weekly basis.

With every breath, you can affirm and anchor the flow of energy as beauty and kindness created within the space of an SEF treatment. Protecting the manifestation of flow is a key to the whole healing process. Learning the skill of protecting the descent of the light of the divine blueprint is equal in importance to the ability to invoke that descent. This teaching is absent in many contemporary schools of healing, including medicine, nursing, massage therapy, herbalism, and energy healing practices. The descent of light that manifests in healing is in direct proportion to the ability of the Partner to hold and garner that light in their spiritual cups—their chakras—and the Provider to prepare and protect the space for that descent. This is the teaching of the purification, protection, and expansion of the auric field. Once energy flows within the body's organs and systems, it becomes an instrument for the radiation of healing light to others. Over time, this energy flow develops a momentum to the point where it opens up and releases like a waterfall. As the chakras are prepared, strengthened, and expanded to be able to hold more light, the Source releases more of that light into the energy field. Both SEF Provider and Partner are engaged in the act of becoming enduring beacons of healing light for humanity. Developing a relationship with this Source of light is like tapping into the fountain of youth. That relationship takes work, devotion, commitment, and constancy. Over time, the fruit of that relationship is recorded as spiritual attainment. The greatest potential of SEF treatment is that it may serve as a platform for the development of a spiritual practice that can ultimately lead to attainment as the active expression of drawing light from the Source in service to humanity. The healing that may come as a result is a gift from that Source and the Creator that comes through the heart of the Provider and the Partner. That is the alchemy or transformational nature of SEF.

Spiritual Protection Practices

In addition to attunement, practices that the Provider engages in at the start of the treatment, some spiritual practices are integral to SEF's transformational nature. Such practices, which can be integrated parts of one's lifestyle, support the creation of that reservoir of light in the aura and chakras to be distributed throughout the nadis, or the channels through which energy flows. Many follow religious practices, some quite ancient, that purify the mind, heart, and emotions. These suggestions are not meant in any way to challenge or replace those practices that provide you with the clarity you seek to be a vessel for healing light. These are simple practices I have picked up during my journey that I consider "tried and true" in terms of attending to the intentions of the SEF Provider who seeks to clear their own energy field of the effluvia that blocks the descent of light from the Source. The ancient Buddhist teachings acknowledge the process of preparation for carrying and protecting the gift:

> *Destroy thy lunar body, cleanse thy mind body and make clean thy heart. Eternal life's pure waters, clear and crystal, with the monsoon tempest's muddy torrents cannot mingle ... The rose must re-become the bud born of its parent stem, before the parasite has eaten through its heart and drunk its life-sap ... Unless the flesh is passive, head cool, the soul as firm and pure as flaming diamond, the radiance will not reach the chamber, its sunlight will not warm the heart, nor will the mystic sounds of the Akasic heights reach the ear, however eager.*[3]

The Healer Jesus gave a key in his teachings to the control of the

---

3 (Blavatsky, 1992 (Originally published in 1889), pp. 11, 17 - 18) The author defines the chamber as the "inner chamber of the Heart, called in Sanskrit *Brahma poori*." The "mystic sounds" or melody is heard at the beginning of a cycle of meditation. (Glossary pages 76 and 78).

energy in the aura when he said, "If therefore thine eye be single, thy whole body shall be full of light." From this, we learn that the light of the body and our energy field is the eye.

At the center of each chakra is a whirling white fire disc of light. Begin by visualizing the white light at the center of your brow, the third eye chakra, as if you were wearing a headlamp as you recite the mantra:

> *Come now by love divine; Guard thou this soul of mine;*
> *Make now my world all thine; God's light around me shine.*
> *(Extend the visualization of white light to fill your auric field.)*
> *I count one; It is done. O feeling world be still.*
> *Two and Three; I AM free; Peace, it is God's will.*
> *(Visualize a band of white fire around the solar plexus nerve center.)*
> *I count four; I do adore my Presence all divine.*
> *Five and six; my God, affix my gaze on thee sublime.*
> *(Visualize a band of white fire around the neck and throat chakra.)*
> *I count seven; Come, O heaven, my energies take hold.*
> *Eight and nine; Completely thine; My mental world enfold.*
> *(Visualize a band of white fire around the head and third eye.)*
> *The white-fire light now encircles me; All riptides are rejected;*
> *With God's own might around me bright; I AM by love protected.*
> *(Visualize white light encircling all of the chakras and the entirety.)*[4]

Place yourself in a position to sit comfortably in a seated meditation posture. As you breathe in and out and allow any tense muscles in your body to soften, fill your awareness with memories and thoughts

---

4   (Djwal Kul & Prophet, 1997 (Originally published in 1974), p. 133)

of love and kindness. Allow your consciousness to sense the sounds, objects, actions, smells, tastes, and sensations that you associate with kindness and its manifestation in daily life.

Maitreya is the name Buddhists associate with the "coming Buddha" whose name is derived from the Sanskrit *maître*, meaning kindness or friendliness. Consider drawing from this ancient Buddhist tradition of kindness meditation and practice to infuse your consciousness with loving kindness. One way to meditate on this is to chant the name of the Buddha whose consciousness you wish to embody. For example, you could chant, "OM - Maitreya - OM." OM or AUM is the ancient sound from which all creation emanates, Alpha to Omega. You can also chant the bija or seed syllable associated with Maitreya. Maitreya's seed syllable is "maim." A seed syllable does not have a meaning per se, but holds spiritual meaning in the sounding of the single syllable. Seed syllables are pronounced as a devotional mantra to a Buddha. There are also other bija mantras that can be chanted to attune with the manifestation of other qualities, such as the wisdom, perseverance, and clear vision of the Dyani Buddhas, who are considered physicians of the soul.

It is also helpful to ask for the assistance of the angels, God's messengers. When I apprenticed with Oma, she taught me one of her daily rituals that she found very helpful in protecting the light released in her foot reflexology work. She asked for the assistance and protection of the seraphim, which are fiery angelic beings. The word seraph means "burning ones." She would pray for them to stand outside the doors to her clinic. It was a free-standing clinic and we would hose down the front of the building with cold water each morning to "demagnetize" the building and then ask the seraphim to stand on both sides of the door. Clients who were sensitive to angelic presence in a space would tell us that they could feel or see the seraphim at work. All that is needed to partner with the seraphim and other angels is a request. Ask them to help and they do, willingly and lovingly. They are kind friends to the SEF Provider who would create a powerful healing environment!

PROMOTING A HEALING ENVIRONMENT

The SEF Provider holds the power of responsibility for creating and sustaining a healing environment for the Partner during the treatment. It is the consciousness of the SEF Provider that first and foremost sets the matrix for the creation of a healing environment. Providers provide not only an environment for the expression of love and wisdom; they also provide power and protection. Sri Aurobindo identified consciousness as power on the yogic path of "man as a transitional being."[5] He wrote,

> It is a mistake of the ethical or religious mind to condemn Power as in itself a thing not to be accepted or sought after because naturally corrupting and evil; in spite of its apparent justification by a majority of instances, this is at its core a blind and irrational prejudice. However corrupted and misused, as Love and Knowledge too are corrupted and misused, Power is divine and put here for a divine use. Shakti, will, Power is the driver of the worlds and whether it be Knowledge-Force or Love-Force or Life-Force or Action-Force or Body-Force, is always spiritual in its origin and divine in its character. It is the use made of it in the Ignorance by brute, man or Titan that has to be cast aside and replaced by its greater natural—even if to us supernormal—action led by an inner consciousness which is in tune with the Infinite and the Eternal. The integral Yoga cannot reject the

---

5   (Satprem & Sri Aurobindo, 1993 (Originally published 1970), p. 235)

188

works of Life and be satisfied with an inward experience only; it has to go inward in order to change the outward.[6]

Sri Aurobindo's teachings seem apropos here because, in particular, he explored the progress that science was making in its work with agni, the term used in ancient Vedic teachings to refer to spiritual fire or power. Specifically, agni is the will in the heart, and that will is the force that dispels ignorance. A healing environment as a co-creation with the Creator for the descent of healing light and under-standing requires power as well as love and wisdom. The external environment is a manifestation of that which is within as love, wisdom, and power. The Provider and the Partner are, in essence, the healing environment. The light and consciousness within is the source of the optimal healing environment that is today so often sought after.[7] Paying attention to the details of the environment without is important to manifesting a healing vibration that is congruent with what is known to be within.

Space, Time, and Effort

Creating a healing environment can be lots of fun as well as a chal-lenge at times. There are three areas to consider when creating an environment in which to conduct the SEF treatment: space, time, and effort. Pay close attention to the physical space. Identify any distrac-tions in the space that will divert your attention from the feet, such as noise (including music), lighting, smells, air quality, wall colors, and "art work." A student of mine was once treating a client in a historic building that had a number of pieces of art on the walls. We set up the treatment table in the most convenient spot in one of the rooms, only to find out that the painting on the wall over the head of the client

---

6   Ibid, p. 232
7   (Jonas & Chez, 2004)

was extremely dark in vibration and, therefore, distracting to both the client and the student. We had to move.

When you design your own space, it is easier to establish a particular healing environment in which to welcome Partners. However, not everyone will find your taste in color, music, or fragrance pleasant, comforting or healing. It is best to be as subtle in fragrance and as neutral and low impact in design as possible to accommodate as many people as you may be helping with your service. You might also consider treating people in their own homes, though that is not without its challenges. Because people's homes are familiar to them, treating them at home holds the potential to diminish the stress associated with being in a new location. This is particularly important when caring for the elderly. Their home is where they feel most secure, particularly if they are suffering from dementia of any kind.

Elders can also be treated in their residential communities. I have also treated people in the hospital when asked to do so. For example, I once had a patient who, upon returning to his hospital room after having a lung removed in surgery, said, "I wish my reflexologist were here. She could help so much with my pain." I told him that I, too, was a reflexologist and he was ecstatic. I gave him a modified post-operative treatment and he slept soundly for hours.

It is also fun to treat people outdoors. Oma and I used to teach large classes in the summer outdoors where people could wade in a cold stream as their footbath before having a foot reflexology treatment. I have also treated people by their pool and at the beach, adapting for sunlight and sand. To treat a Partner in their home or outdoors, you will need a "go bag." I have a canvas duffel bag that holds my footbath basin, towels, pack materials, oils, and client files so that I can be ready to take SEF with me on any call to help someone. You will also need a portable table or chair. I use a portable, light-weight, zero-gravity folding chair that allows me to give the Partner their footbath in a seated position and then shift them back in the chair so that I can lift their feet up and lay them back into a reclined position for the treatment and pack. The only space that this requires is enough room for the folding chair and three additional feet around the chair to accommodate yourself and your supplies. As the Provider, you can sit on a rolling stool, which can be moved easily out of the way when you stand to apply the pack.

Time is another factor in creating a healing environment. An SEF treatment with footbath and pack takes approximately 45 minutes; however, you can decide with your Partner whether to provide a footbath or leave the pack in place for a longer time. It is best to agree on these details before starting the treatment so that expectations are managed and the treatment can flow smoothly from the preparation phase to sealing. Be aware that the recommended amount of time for the SEF treatment should include the time needed to ring the bells and address the entirety. Do not linger on any partic-ular point or system. Move through the treatment of the entirety as quickly as possible.

Ultimately, the goal of the Provider in an SEF treatment is to move effortlessly through the treatment whether sitting or standing, applying a pack or kneeling before the Partner while washing their feet. One way to determine the amount of effort being used is to monitor the use of your shoulders! Stand in front of a mirror and look at the space between your ear lobes and the top of your shoulders. You can even measure the distance with a tape measure. Take a deep breath and drop your shoulders. Push your hand down your side as you push your shoulder down. When your shoulders are raised, then you are not in position to treat efficiently. Your shoulders should be dropped and then your elbow and/or wrist should be raised or lowered to accommodate the proper thumb or finger position on the foot. If you find that you are straining in a particular position or unable to work an energy field as described in this book, try adjusting your shoulders first. Place your hands in front of you again and look at your natural hand and thumb placement. Then go back to the feet and start in that position of natural alignment. Effortless SEF moves from the center of the body, the heart and the core. Dropping the shoulders and using natural hand placement becomes effortless when used as the point of reference for the work.

The other energetic contribution to the effort or effortlessness of a treatment has to do with the preparation and consciousness of the Partner. What is the investment of the Partner in the treatment? Have they initiated the treatment or did a friend or family member? Or did you suggest it? If so, the effort expended in the treatment may be exponential as compared with the person who has a tremendous interest in the SEF treatment, has read a little bit about it (looked at the chart or this book, for example), and has talked about their desire for treatment. While I do support the use of SEF in the home, particularly for the elderly as I stated, I also realize the importance of a person making an effort that expends some amount of energy to put them in a position to receive an SEF treatment. I have often had to make a tremendous effort to place myself in a position to receive a healing. I recently experienced a deep inner healing when I traveled thousands of miles to New Zealand. In many traditions, a journey or pilgrimage is part of the healing process. Qigong master Ken Cohen writes, "Sometimes, it is the patient who must make a pilgrimage to aid in his or her own healing, perhaps to gather a medicinal plant or commune with a healing power. The very act of traveling to a new landscape helps us release unhealthy habits and opens the mind to unexpected vistas. We can make a pilgrimage more healing and rewarding by celebrating the landscape, a custom of indigenous people throughout the world."[8] I agree. This is another reason that I have positioned my professional SEF practice at a hospital center with a labyrinth where my clients can take a "journey" walking in their Swedish Bitters packs. I often give "homework" like this to my clients so that they never slip into the mode of passive recipient of SEF or any of the cares provided to assist in their healing work. SEF, in lay or professional practice, is really a support to Self-care, the journey to understanding the elements of Self as described throughout this book.

PROFESSIONAL PRACTICE AND SEF

The focus of this book is to describe and define SEF as it can be practiced in self-care and in the assistance of family and friends at home and in community. It also can be an integrated part of professional health care practice. For nearly 30 years, it has been a joy for me to apply SEF in my service as a registered and then advanced practice nurse. SEF foot reflexology effects measurable positive change in people's health. As a researcher, I find positive correlations between SEF treatments and changes in health patterns. I have trained hundreds of professionals who are licensed to touch (physicians, nurses, massage, and body workers, for example) how they, too, can integrate SEF foot reflexology in their practice plans. Those who hold licenses in any health care practice and who wish to provide professional-level SEF treatment and charge for it as a service and practice modality for their clients/ patients have additional considerations and responsibilities.

First, read the legal documents that guide your scope of practice for which you are licensed. Become aware of how reflexology and foot reflexology are regulated—if at all. Typically, specific names of

---

8   (Cohen, 2003, p. 68)

therapies are not included in a Practice Act because there are simply too many to name. Generally speaking, a Practice Act will require a licensee to be educated in the modalities they employ in their practice. Those modalities must also fit within the defined Scope of Practice for that license. Foot reflexology is a touch therapy and, therefore, a person wishing to provide professional-level foot reflexology must be licensed to touch. Practice Acts are written with the safety of the public in mind. Foot reflexology as a touch modality is fundamentally safe in that it is non-invasive and stress-reducing. What opponents of the work have historically cited in publication as the biggest safety issues are concerns about the diagnostic validity (of foot reflexology charts)[9] and claims made about the therapeutic effects of the modality.

If a practitioner uses a foot reflexology chart or treatment to diagnose medical disease—even if they are licensed to do so—there is a professional "culture clash." Diseases are diagnostic patterns constructed according to a specific paradigm, the biomedical paradigm. Foot reflexology is anchored squarely in a paradigm related to energy flow, not biomedical disease identification. Therefore, foot reflexology charts should never be used to diagnose the diseases of the biomedical paradigm. While I may be licensed to diagnose depression, for example, I do not diagnose "depression" from the feet. However, because foot reflexology diagnostics are related to energy flow, I may find blockages of energy flow in the liver, an organ typically associated with depression in Traditional Chinese Medicine, for example.

The distinction between the biomedical paradigm and energetic views described in detail in this book suggests that those who practice foot reflexology learn new language for describing the effects of foot reflexology. Any description of the effects of foot reflexology—that is, any claims about its effects on health—must be relayed in energetic

---

9   (White, Williamson, Hart, & Ernst, 2000)

terms rather than biomedical diagnostic or therapeutic terms. When this clear focus is maintained about the science, art, and effects of foot reflexology, all of the opposing arguments become nil. The science of energy flow, as it is practiced in the art of foot reflexology, is an energetic touch therapy with deep historical roots. All attempts to biomedicalize the modality undermine the momentum of safe practice, as the tradition has been handed down from generation to generation. All attempts to define the effects of foot reflexology or destroy its record of safety and credibility as a healing science and art in biomedical terms fail to reach the mark when the focus remains energy flow.

Energy flow is not the specified domain of any one particular health care practice or any human endeavor, for that matter. Some might say that demonstrating knowledge of energy flow is the right and fundamental responsibility of all human endeavors. In fact, if health practitioners are to individualize care, they must be free to address the unique, energetic needs of every individual client. Protection of public safety in the realm of health care relies on the freedom to individualize care. Many biomedical-based clinicians find SEF classes to support the direction they have been seeking to provide individualized care. The SEF courses teach the ability to define, diagnose, and treat energy flow as a health pattern through the application of specific touch skills to the entirety represented in the feet.

Science of Energy Flow® Foot Reflexology is a protected registered trademark of Golden Apple Healing Arts. To advertise professional practice of Science of Energy Flow® Foot Reflexology requires two certificates of course completion, one for the SEF Level 1 introductory class with an SEF-certified teacher and one for Level 2 Apprenticeship. There are two levels for certificate completion. Level 1 is at least a 30-hour, introductory hands-on workshop and the second level is a two-day workshop followed by a distance-learning apprenticeship of case and practice review. All of the skills outlined in this book are requirements for certification and use of the Science of Energy Flow® Foot Reflexology title. A requirement of Science of Energy Flow® Foot Reflexology certification is that all practitioners, regardless of biomedical diagnostic ability, must be able to perform energetic pattern recognition analyses and treatment of the feet. This book is the textbook for that training.

Professional practitioners also are responsible for staying informed as to the state of the science and current research on foot reflexology, hydrotherapy footbaths, and topical herbal applications used in SEF. They must also accurately measure and report outcomes of foot reflexology treatments. When possible, SEF and foot reflexology practitioners make contributions to the scientific advancement of these modalities. One way to do this is by conducting regular literature searches in PUBMED, the database of the United States National Library of Medicine. By using the clinical queries function, practitioners can quickly retrieve a very organized dataset on a subject such as foot reflexology.[10] Another excellent Web-based resource for foot reflexology research is reflexologists Barbara and Kevin Kunz's Reflexology Research Project.[11]

There is a body of biomedical research on foot reflexology that dates back to the 1990s, if not before. One of the first foot reflexology studies I became aware of was published in 1993. The study, a randomized controlled trial, suggested a decrease in premenstrual symptoms for women given "true" reflexology treatments as compared with those in the placebo group.[12] A true reflexology treatment in this study

---

10   http://www.ncbi.nlm.nih.gov/pubmed/clinical
11   http://www.reflexology-research.com
12   (Oleson & Flocco, 1993)

included manual pressure to specific points: ovary, uterus, pituitary gland, adrenal gland, kidney, solar plexus, and sympathetic nervous system. Specific points in the ear and hand were also worked in the treatment group. The "placebo" group was given "uneven tactile stimulation to areas of the ears, hands, and feet considered inappropriate for menstrual problems such as the nose, shoulder, and abdomen.[13] This a good example of some of the concerns in applying quantitative research designs when inquiring about the nature of ancient treatments such as reflexology. In order to apply an experimental design in which numerous variables are controlled, the researchers must remove the scientific and cultural contexts that have supported the use of the tradition in the healing arts for centuries. The removal of these contexts typically results in a significant change in the modality and the tradition. The question then raised is whether the study is measuring the actual effect of the modality or simply some aspect of the modality.

Despite the efforts of many practitioners and researchers, there are some gaps that remain between clinical practice and research.[14] Part of the reasons for these gaps has to do with culture clash. Some within the dominant biomedical culture either knowingly or unknowingly impose scientific views, which are culturally derived, on all research, often calling for randomized controlled trials (RCTs). These RCTs are sometimes done with the purpose of debunking "anecdotal or unpublished claims" of those who practice and would "mislead the public."[15] The RCT, however, is just one of many research designs that can help further the understanding of modalities such as foot reflexology. Designing an RCT, which is an experimental design, requires lots of

---

13   Ibid p. 908
14   (Tonelli, 1998)
15   (Wilkinson & Rayner, 2003, p. 98)

control in an effort to show causation between the intervention (foot reflexology) and an outcome or change in human behavior. RCTs also involve placebos, which have been shown in actual studies to be as much as 40 percent effective[16] in relieving symptoms of diseases such as depression, hypertension, and asthma.

Other designs, such as correlational studies, do not require such rigorous control. Such a design in quantitative research is commonly used for those phenomena that cannot or should not be controlled, as would an experimental design. Correlational studies seek to understand relationships rather than causation. Reflexologists and the public could benefit from evidence born of correlational studies and qualitative studies as well. People seek to know "how" as well as "why" reflexology treatments seem to effect a change in symptoms or energy flow. Whatever the research method used, a "true" study would examine reflexology with interventions that reflect the modality as it is within its traditional and historical clinical context rather than measuring an adapted version that fits into the mold for a particular study design.

If foot reflexology were viewed simply as the pushing of points, then an RCT might well be feasible. But as Oma once said, "Foot reflexology is not the pushing of points." The quest for knowledge or the use of a modality should not rise and fall on whether or not that modality can be studied according to the tenets of the science that values the RCT. Proper research should be conducted in a way that systematically examines the question without bias as to any pre-chosen method or design. There are those who demonstrate prejudice against complementary therapies such as reflexology simply because the modality does not meet their biomedical worldview and, not surprisingly, is unable to be measured by the RCTs and statistics

---

16   (Brown, 1998; Walach & Jonas, 2004)

held as the "gold standard" of science.[17] There are, in fact, studies that do follow research standards that find support for the use of reflexology or some version of it in the alleviation of pain and symptoms of disease or, at the very least, add to the understanding of some aspect of the science of reflexology.[18]

These are all common issues of scientific research in general and not necessarily a reflection on the nature of any one particular treatment. If a treatment were barred from being applied and reviewed by an individual clinician simply because of a dearth of RCTs, one would wonder what physicians would do every day in their practices. A study by the U.S. Office of Technology Assessment (1998) recorded that only 20 percent of treatments used in medical care had been subjected to "empirical trials" and shown to be effective.[19] This is understandable when one realizes that some questions do not lend themselves to RCTs, and the time and cost involved in carrying out a single RCT to completion is very high. Dr. C. Everett Koop, as Surgeon General of the United States from 1982 to 1989, questioned the affordability and sustainability of the American health care system that values the RCT so greatly as opposed to inviting all ways of knowing. According to Koop, "It may be possible that in the new millennium, we may be more ready to ask the peoples of the developing world to share their wisdom with us."[20] His prediction has been on target.[21]

---

17   (Wang, Tsai, Lee, Chang, & Yang, 2008; White et al., 2000)
18   (Nakamaru, Miura, Fukushima, & Kawashima, 2008; Siev-Ner, Gamus, Lerner-Geva, & Achiron, 2003; Stephenson, Weinrich, & Tavakoli, 2000)
19   (Brown, 1998, p. 90)
20   (Micozzi, 1996, pp. x-xi)
21   See www.bamboobridge.org

EVOLUTION OF ENTIRETY

Wisdom is knowledge in practice, over time. Working the entirety in SEF is wisdom. To reduce a foot treatment to the pushing of one point or set of points representing an organ, body systems, or energy field goes against the underlying philosophy of wholeness that is the entirety. The entirety must be treated to be an SEF treatment. The rationale and insight for this wisdom is demonstrated in this book; however, there are occasions in the treatment of certain types of energy patterns that manifest in a particular type of client during which one can observe themes that develop between the treatments that clients with similar health concerns receive. While the entirety is treated in all clients, certain health patterns in different individuals may take on similar strengths. Some of those treatment themes are presented in the next section for your review.

Treatment Themes – Health Patterns and Disease

Stuffy Sinuses

One of the most physical responses people seem to have to SEF is the clearance of their sinuses, particularly when the sinuses are milked and the head area is worked. When a person talks about stuffy sinuses, suggest a Chamomile footbath and SEF. Chamomile flower has anti-inflammatory properties and, when inhaled during a footbath, soothes the sinuses and helps release stuffiness.

Self-Limited Disease

"Self-limited disease" is a historic term defined by Dr. Jacob Bigelow, a medical leader during the nineteenth-century health care reform period in America, as a disease that "receives limits from its own nature, and not from foreign influences; one which, after it has obtained foothold in the system, cannot, in the present state of our knowledge, be eradicated, or abridged, by art,—but to which there is due a certain succession of processes, to be completed in a certain time; which time and processes may vary with the constitution and condition of the patient, and may tend to death, or to recovery, but are not known to be shortened, or greatly changed, by medical treatment."[22] An example of a self-limited disease is the common cold. Excessive stress is a known challenge to the immune system. Prior to an SEF treatment, ask the client to rate their overall stress level on a scale from 1 to 10 (10 is a high level of stress and 1 is little to no stress). Ask them the same question after the SEF treatment as well. SEF treatments effectively reduce clients' perception of negative stress. It can be hypothesized that any treatment that supports the natural immune response to the common cold or any self-limited disease might increase client comfort and perseverance while the disease is running its natural self-limited course. A "tincture of time (Thyme)" is often helpful during cold and flu season. Thyme herb or bath oil used in footbaths can permeate the healing environment with anti-microbial molecules and the essence of a plant that strengthens the thymus gland or heart chakra. Tapping the sternum under which the thymus gland is located may help in the process of promoting an immune response[23] that supports the process of self-limitation.

Post-Partum Care for Mothers and Infants

One of the most important times for health promotion in the life of any person is during the first days after birth. Bonding, adjustment, adaptation, and movement or energy flow support the health develop-

---

22   (Bigelow, 1836, p. 8)

23   (Libster, 2012, pp. 409-410)

ment of a newborn infant and the healthy return of a mother's body to a pre-pregnancy state. Breastfeeding is one of the most important health behaviors that provide that necessary support for healthy infants and mothers. Breastfeeding is the result of energy flow, the flow of milk. I have used SEF very successfully with moms and babies after birth to assist in the breastfeeding and bonding processes. Some moms, particularly new moms, experience a goodly amount of stress regarding their ability to successfully breastfeed their infants. Footbaths and SEF treatments assist in stress reduction and often result in activation of the let-down response (the flow of breast milk), particularly if the baby is nearby when the mom receives her treatment. As the mom relaxes in the footbath and the Provider touches the feet, energy flows downward. The mom who has been holding her baby inside her body and maintaining an upright posture begins to shift her weight back to pre-pregnancy stance with the activation of proprioceptive centers in the feet during SEF. The mom and baby are in heightened states of awareness so as to be sensitive to each other's non-verbal cues; so it is important for the SEF Provider to remember that the energy fields for the various chakras, organs, and systems will be very close to the surface. Those whose hands are trained and sensitive to energy flow will find that ringing the bell requires little to no pressure as the fields are close to the surface of the feet. For those who are in training, it is best to practice simply touching the points in post-partum women and infants and doing the visualizations as described. The entire treatment is essentially made up of calming touches and holds. The natural intensity of life force does the rest of the balancing and re-balancing very nicely with support from SEF. Infants' energy fields remain on the surface for some months, typically until they start to creep or crawl. My treatments of infants are fondly referred to as "beep" treatments. They are quick, light, and follow the baby's natural movement responding to their change in position during the SEF treatment. Infants do not typi-cally need to receive footbaths or packs. Rose infused oil is the preferred oil for anointing the feet as the Rose oil provides protection to the baby's nervous system as it anchors more fully in the physical plane. However, be very careful about using any fragrance or odors—even the smells of medicinal-grade essential oils in the space where the baby and mom are treated often disrupt physical and spiritual attachments (including breastfeeding) forming between the mother and baby.

Diabetes

Foot care is part of routine medical care of the diabetic patient; however, diabetic foot care focuses on nail trimming and skin care. Imagine what might happen if those who provide diabetic foot care also gave SEF treatments! Foot reflexology is standard care in China for diabetic patients and has been studied extensively.[24] SEF foot reflexology, in particular, holds tremendous potential for assisting the diabetic client in managing the health patterns associated with their disease as well as their skin. Castor oil packs keep the skin of the feet moist and supple.

Cancer Treatment Support

One of the hardest times for people undergoing cancer treatment is when they experience the severe nausea that often happens due to chemotherapy treatment. Vomiting, or reflux of qi, is viewed in Traditional Chinese Medicine as the body's way of dealing with stagnation of energy or blocked energy flow. When the energy in the digestive organs, stomach, gallbladder, liver, and small intestine does not flow through the proper channels, it refluxes or moves in a

24   http://www.reflexology-research.com

different direction. Nausea and vomiting are some of the results of what is essentially a normal adaptation response. Citrus peel is one herb that moves qi in the abdomen. SEF also assists in unblocking energy. SEF treatment with an anointing blend that includes sweet orange essential oil can be considered for cancer patients undergoing chemotherapy. I created a program for the University of Colorado Cancer Center in which members of the team taught patients' care-givers to give a basic foot massage with citrus massage oil. The foot massages were often very effective in helping energy move during the chemotherapy experience.

Stroke

My Norwegian teacher Charles was particularly interested in helping people who had suffered stroke. He applied Foot Zone Therapy treatments with amazing results in which stroke symptoms, such as aphasia, resolved after treatments. As stated here, he stressed and taught me the importance of always treating the "entirety." But there is a difference in intention when working with stroke victims that should be mentioned. Be sure to focus on the proper physiology when holding the vision for this patient's healing. Strokes in the left side of the brain cause right-sided symptoms and vice versa. Therefore, when working the great toe on each foot, be sure to visualize the healing and wholeness for the proper side of the body related to the toe you are working on. Anoint the feet with St. John's Wort infused oil and work the feet through before applying a Castor oil pack. St. John's Wort flowers and buds heal wounds and nerves.

Adoption and Birth Trauma

Many illnesses, stressors, and diseases are the ultimate manifestation of the spiritual distress and emotional pain or trauma experienced around the time of birth and infancy. Adoption, the separation from one's biological parents, is one such example of birth crisis. Upon examining a history of birth crises, we often find that the person has not fully embodied or taken "root" in their body. Over the years, I have had the opportunity to help many children whose health patterns suggest that they have not fully embodied. For example, they may be prone to injury, unaware of where they are in space. They may be very psychic or highly sensitive to the environment. Some children become mentally ill, even psychotic. The SEF foot reflexology treatments help children to anchor themselves in their bodies. The feet are our roots. The herbal packs and oils help their nervous systems to heal, release any imperil, and then allow for the soul to come more fully into their own being. This is very important in children who have been adopted. I have cared for children who start to have memories of their birth parents and become very uncomfortable in their bodies as a result. SEF creates an environment for work on the under-standing. As the children relax, they work with their adoptive parents and counselors to find solutions to sorting out their feelings and relationships.

Pain and Inflammation

An SEF treatment given in concert with a fresh Ginger compress to the kidneys can be very helpful in reducing pain and inflammation that may be local or systemic.

HOW TO PERFORM A GINGER COMPRESS

Grate 4 to 5 ounces (150 g) of fresh Ginger root. Put the Ginger into a small cloth bag and add it to 1 gallon (3.8 liters) of simmering (not boiling) water. Allow the decoction to steep gently for 5 minutes. Holding both ends of a hand towel, dip the middle of the towel into the Ginger water. Wring it out and fold it to the size of the client's mid-back where the kidneys are. Take care in applying the hot compress, making sure that the skin does not burn because of the heat. The compress should be applied as hot as is tolerated. Place a dry towel over the compress and a blanket over the towel, tucking each layer around the client so that air does not enter the compress and cool it. Prepare a second compress as the first. Replace the first compress after 3 to 4 minutes. Remove the blanket and dry towel. Place the second hot compress on top of the first and flip the compress over, making sure that the temperature is tolerated. This technique ensures that the connection with the Ginger and moist heat is maintained. The compresses should be flipped every 3 to 4 minutes for 20 minutes. The Ginger compress will create increased circulation of blood and body fluids, and move qi and blood stagnation that usually manifests as pain, inflammation, swelling, or stiffness. Many people with chronic pain benefit from Ginger compresses to the kidneys as a systemic remedy rather than the application of compresses to individual joints. Ginger compresses should not be used when high fever is present (too warming), on the head area, on the abdomen in pregnancy, for infants or the very old (too stimulating), or on an area of the body experiencing infection (heat), such as the chest/lung area during pneumonia.

Difficulty Breathing

When difficult breathing is determined to be non-life threatening but deeply stressful, as is often the case in those with chronic lung disease, SEF treatments can be very helpful in releasing the stress in the diaphragm muscle and solar plexus nerve center (See Solar Plexus hold and treatment). Take care when using any essential oils as these clients' respiratory systems may react strongly to certain odors or substances. With asthma, the client has difficulty exhaling, a condition referred to in Traditional Chinese Medicine as lungs not "grasping qi." SEF treatments break the respiratory pattern of excessive inhalation and locked chest without exhalation so that a normal rhythm with the rise and fall of the chest can return. The Castor oil packs are very soothing to the nervous system and calming to the person who may be anxious due to the inability to exhale fully.

Constipation

The SEF footbath and treatment draw the energy to and through the feet. Constipation is relieved when the large intestine empties properly. Stress, diet, lifestyle (such as lack of sleep), and disease can all point to a propensity for chronic constipation. Acute constipation can occur after surgical procedures or other traumas to the body. During trauma, energy shifts to the more critical life-sustaining organs, such as the heart and lungs, and away from the intestines. Decreasing the stress response signals the body that the crisis is over and bowel function can return to normal. This process takes time. SEF footbath and treatment can help to decrease the stress response and move energy in the large intestine. At one hospital where I worked as a new graduate nurse, I was known for my ability to help post-operative patients get discharged sooner because I would put their feet in a footbath and give them a foot massage. That alone gets the bowels moving. Given the fact that the large intestine covers all 10 zones of the body, it is imperative to be able to keep the energy flowing in that organ.

Mental and Spiritual Distress

When people become mentally or spiritually distressed, they often start to spin. SEF treatments help people to under-stand the importance of stopping the spinning by centering, visualizing wholeness, and protecting and healing the nervous system. Sipping Lemongrass

DR. MARTHA'S OATMEAL COOKIE RECIPE

Ingredients:
¾ cup butter, softened
1 cup packed brown sugar
½ cup granulated sugar
1 teaspoon baking powder
¼ teaspoon baking soda
½ teaspoon ground Cinnamon (optional)
¼ teaspoon ground Cloves (optional)
¼ teaspoon ground Lemongrass
¼ teaspoon ground Coriander
2 eggs
1 teaspoon Vanilla
1¾ cups all-purpose flour
2 cups rolled oats

Directions:
Preheat oven to 375 degrees F/190 degrees C. In a large mixing bowl, beat butter with an electric mixer on medium to high speed for 30 seconds. Add brown sugar, granulated sugar, baking powder, baking soda, and spices. Beat until combined, scraping side of bowl occasionally. Beat in eggs and vanilla until combined. Beat in as much of the flour as you can with the mixer. Using a wooden spoon, stir in any remaining flour. Stir in rolled oats. Drop dough by rounded teaspoons 2 inches apart onto ungreased cookie sheets. Bake for 8 to 10 minutes or until edges are golden. Let stand on cookie sheets for 1 minute. Transfer to wire racks and let cool. Makes about 48 cookies.

tea is a calming complement to an SEF treatment for those in distress. The grass grows straight and has a light, uplifting smell. I serve homemade oatmeal cookies with the Lemongrass tea. Oats are also calming to the nervous system. After providing the SEF treatment, Lemongrass tea, and oatmeal cookies, I recommend that the client get a full night's sleep. I then check on the client in the morning. It is amazing what a great effect sleep can have on relieving distress.

Couples and Family
(Emotional Distress and Miscommunication)

One of the best therapies for couples and families experiencing emotional distress and miscommunication in their relationships is an SEF footbath. Miscommunication and strong emotions do not typically last long in the space of the foot washing. It is hard to be angry at someone who is kneeling at your feet washing them in a soothing footbath. Children love to help their families during times of distress. An SEF footbath is a healing act that they are often very good at that decreases stress levels and increases healing.

Sleep

SEF treatments are often best offered in the evening for those who are having trouble sleeping. SEF allows the client to sink into a very restful state. The hot footbath and Castor oil packs are very helpful in facilitating sound sleep. Do not apply a Swedish Bitters pack before sleep for those who are having trouble sleeping.

Death and Transition

SEF treatments are an excellent therapy for those preparing for death. Family members who know how to give an SEF footbath and treatment often comment how helpful it was to be able to provide comfort for their loved one who was making the transition. Consider providing sips of Flat Leaf Parsley and/or Lemon Balm tea for the person before and after the treatment. These two plants help to deal with excess uric acid in the body that often causes pain. Parsley tea is a traditional remedy that helps the kidneys during the death transition. Lemon Balm lifts the spirit as the SEF treatment eases the person's burden in the feet and they become lighter.

CONCLUSION – SEF AND HEALTH CARE REFORM

As the feet receive SEF treatments over time, they and their energy field—the entirety—become filled with light. How and when this actually occurs is perhaps best described as a "gift." That gift represents all the good work, effort, visualization, and drawing down of the matrix of wholeness, ultimately described as attainment. Attainment is an anchor of light in one's spiritual body registered as memory much the way a passing grade is recorded by a teacher after scoring an examination. Once the lesson is learned, the attainment released is like a key that unlocks a door. The door opens to a waterfall of light, the movement of which is flow. With every key or passing grade, the momentum of light becomes stronger; energy flow becomes stronger.

This is why the primary focus of SEF foot reflexology is the spinning of the chakras by activating the energy fields of the associated glands. The Tau Spiral meditation prepares the chakras to act as cups that will hold the light as it descends from the blueprint of wholeness. The white light in the core center of each chakra represents the complete cycle of energy Alpha to Omega, the beginning and the ending, the whirling Tai Chi. Just as with every recitation of the ancient sound AUM, every successive treatment strengthens the chakras and the energy field through the flow of energy Alpha to Omega. The physical manifestation of this anchoring of attainment of energy flow is through close, mindful observation of individual health patterns. An experienced eye can detect in the health pattern the growing ability to sustain and maintain health and well being for longer periods of time without impediments from within or without. Co-creation of Self with God the Creator gradually replaces all illusion. Each experience of the grace of God the Creator as the descent of healing light brings greater balance, understanding of one's true nature and, thus, the gradual and permanent dissolution of all desire for material gain as human greed that blocks energy flow. SEF is just the kind of treatment modality needed at this time when people are calling for health care reform. What is needed is SEF with its tried-and-true enduring momentum of healing tradition backed by ancient wisdom.

People cry out in their souls for health care reform. This is not a new phenomenon; it was one of the primary social objectives of the early and mid-nineteenth century in the United States before the Civil War. I have researched and written on the role of nurses during that social period.[25] It was a time during which people highly valued "Being Their Own Doctor." Not unlike today, numerous books about self-care and home remedies and treatments permeated the market-place. These texts were referred to as "domestic medicine" guides and "advice books." Their contents typically included instruction on the care of the sick as well as on promoting health. The management of the sick room and preparation of diets for the sick were outlined in detail and included the regulation of the natural elements ether, fire (heat), air, water, and earth. People treated their health concerns with

---

25   (Libster, 2004; Libster & McNeil, 2009)

modified versions of therapeutics that had been used for centuries, such as water or hydrotherapies and herbal remedies. There was a tiered system of health care at that time. The first tier involved self-care—providing care for oneself and one's family. People perceived that they were qualified, with the support of knowledgeable community healers, to assess the nature and severity of their own health concerns and devise ways to relieve their discomfort and promote health. When they needed more help because their pain did not go away or their concern for their condition grew, they sought the help of another more knowledgeable community member. In the nineteenth century, that helper might be a hydrotherapist known as a "water curist" or an herbalist, a midwife, bonesetter, homeopath, surgeon, physician, or a nurse. But health care began at home and, therefore, health care reform began at home. And so it is today.

Health care reform begins at home. It begins with each one of us. This book, Science of Energy Flow®, is about a modality that can be readily applied and how each person becomes the health care-reformed nation we seek because health care reform is not only about resource management. It is most certainly not only about management of medical resources in hospitals and doctor's offices, which is the primary focus of most of the political dialog for the past decades. Health care reform involves change, and that change over time means evolution of the elements of Self as physical, mental, emotional, and spiritual beings.

The notions of reform and evolution—personal, in community, and as a nation—are defined within the context of history rather than in the present moment in which we live. We enter into the process with faith, hope, and charity and realize that the outcome is not completely within our control. The outer manifestation of health care reform and evolution draws upon:

- Health freedom - the right to choose how to heal and to be one's own healer
- Health literacy - the knowledge to be one's own healer
- Health belief - the inner conviction to be one's own healer

The inner manifestation of health care reform and evolution is demonstrated in healing service to humanity. SEF Foot Reflexology with Herbal Stress Relief, as described in this little book, is a platform for both the outer and inner manifestations of reform and evolution. It is a healing modality for the twenty-first century when the light that flows from the feet to the brain, sending a signal for the release of a wholeness current, not only radiates love, wisdom, and power to one's own body, but also blesses and comforts all life with the purity of the same. This is my vision of the future of the healing arts.

I end this book with a final note of encouragement to you who would take on this work of reform and evolution. Guard your heart. Do your own ablutions every day and anoint your hands at the end of each day of helping others with the purest Rose oil you can find Massage that Rose oil into your solar plexus and your feet as you breathe deeply and visualize the violet fire passing through your body to transmute any and all negative energy and imperil you may have taken in. Keep your peace and let no one ever take your joy! The healing arts have forever been a joyful path.

SEF is a joyful path to walk in beauty. I see my clients walking their path of beauty after an SEF treatment in winged sandals. That was a vision I was shown by an angel many years ago at the end of a treatment. While gently patting the feet, I saw the sandals appear at inner planes on the feet and heard a clapping sound that I recognized as the gentle beating together of angels' wings. In that moment, I realized that the joy of SEF is shared not only between Providers and

Partners, but with the angels as well. They clap their wings for every successful SEF treatment accomplished. They clap now that I have told you this story, for they know that what one can do, all can do and that as each person—foot by foot—is treated, everyone is touched by the flow of healing energy.

Bigelow, J. (1836). "Discourse on Self-Limited Disease." *Medical Communications of the Massachusetts Medical Society*. Boston: The Massachusetts Medical Society.

Blavatsky, H. (1992 (Originally published in 1889)). *The Voice of the Silence: Being Chosen Fragments from the 'Book of the Golden Precepts.'* Pasadena, California: Theosophical University Press.

Brown, W. A. (1998). "The Placebo Effect." *Scientific American*, 278(1), 90-95.

Cohen, K. (2003). "Where Healing Dwells: The Importance of Sacred Space." *Alternative Therapies in Health and Medicine*, 9(4), 68-72.

Djwal Kul, & Prophet, E. C. (1997 (Originally published in 1974)). *Intermediate Studies of the Human Aura*. Los Angeles, California: Summit University Press.

Jonas, W. B., & Chez, R. A. (2004). "Toward Optimal Healing Environments in Health Care." *Journal of Alternative and Complementary Medicine*, 10 Suppl 1, S1-6.

Libster, M. (2004). *Herbal Diplomats: The Contribution of Early American Nurses (1830-1860) to Nineteenth-Century Health Care Reform and the Botanical Medical Movement*. http://www.GoldenApplePublications.com: Golden Apple Publications.

Libster, M. (2012). *The Nurse-Herbalist: Integrative Insights for Holistic Practice*. http://www.Goldenapplepublications.com: Golden Apple Publications.

Libster, M., & McNeil, B. A. (2009). *Enlightened Charity: The Holistic Nursing Care, Education and Advices Concerning the Sick of Sister Matilda Coskery, (1799-1870)*. http://www.GoldenAppleHealingArts.com: Golden Apple Publications.

Micozzi, M. (1996). *Fundamentals of Complementary and Alternative Medicine*. New York: Churchill Livingstone Inc.

Nakamaru, T., Mlura, N., Fukushima, A., & Kawashima, R. (2008). "Somatotopical Relationships between Cortical Activity and Reflex Areas in Reflexology: A Functional Magnetic Resonance Imaging Study." *Neuroscience Letters*, 448(1), 6-9.

Oleson, T., & Flocco, W. (1993). "Randomized Controlled Study of Premenstrual Symptoms Treated with Ear, Hand, and Foot Reflexology." *Obstetrics & Gynecology*, 82(6), 906-911.

Roerich, H. (1929). *Agni Yoga*. New York: Agni Yoga Society.

Satprem, & Sri Aurobindo. (1993 (Originally published 1970)). *Sri Aurobindo, or The Adventure of Consciousness*. New York: Institute for Evolutionary Research.

Siev-Ner, I., Gamus, D., Lerner-Geva, L., & Achiron, A. (2003). "Reflexology Treatment Relieves Symptoms of Multiple Sclerosis: A Randomized Controlled Study." *Multiple Sclerosis*, 9(4), 356-361.

Stephenson, N. L., Weinrich, S. P., & Tavakoli, A. S. (2000). "The Effects of Foot Reflexology on Anxiety and Pain in Patients with Breast and Lung Cancer." *Oncology Nursing Forum*, 27(1), 67-72.

Tonelli, M. (1998). "The Philosophical Limits of Evidence-based Medicine." *Academic Medicine*, 73(12), 1234-1240.

Walach, H., & Jonas, W. (2004). "Placebo Research: The Evidence Base for Harnessing Self-healing Capacities." *Journal of Alternative and Complementary Medicine, 10 Suppl 1*, S103-112.

Wang, M.-Y., Tsai, P.-S., Lee, P.-H., Chang, W.-Y., & Yang, C.-M. (2008). "The Efficacy of Reflexology: Systematic Review." *Journal of Advanced Nursing*, 62(5), 512-520.

White, A. R., Williamson, J., Hart, A., & Ernst, E. (2000). "A Blinded Investigation into the Accuracy of Reflexology Charts." *Complementary Therapies in Medicine*, 8(3), 166-172.

Wilkinson, I., & Rayner, C. (2003). "Letter to the Editor: The Future of Reflexology." *Complementary Therapies in Nursing and Midwifery*, 9(2), 98.

Summary of Basic Treatment

SCIENCE OF ENERGY FLOW®
FOOT REFLEXOLOGY WITH HERBAL STRESS RELIEF

1. Attunement - Centering - Light as Energy Flow!

2. Ablution - Five element footbaths and "washing" of the feet.

    Invoking violet fire.

3. Anointing - Work the feet through with natural oil blend

    Always have both hands on one foot. Either both hands are working at the same time or one is holding the foot while the other is working. Work from the palms of the hands rather than from the fingertips.

4. Approach -

    • Work the sinus areas to open them.

    • Initial motions: holds, positions, techniques.

    • Solar plexus hold and treatment.

        Hold each solar plexus point with one thumb.

        Eight-part breathing with client to relax diaphragm and solar plexus:

        1. Breathe in for eight counts.

        2. Suspend breath for eight counts.

        3. Breathe out for eight counts.

        4. Hold out for eight counts.

        5. Repeat using visualization.

5. Tau Spiral chakra meditation –

    Activate endocrine gland energy fields:

    Start with the thymus, then thyroid, adrenals, pineal, pancreas, pituitary, ovaries/testes/uterus.

    Chakra visualization.

6. Step-by-step work through all systems:

    Lymphatic system.

    Spine walking and joints.

    Respiratory system.

    Gastrointestinal system.

    Urinary system.

7. Sealing of the feet and herbal stress relief:

    Wrap or pack.

    Walk the spine with a drop of Mint essential oil.

    Sealing.

INDEX

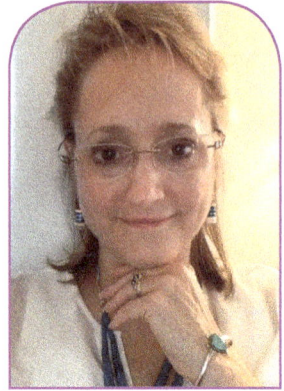

DR. MARTHA MATHEWS LIBSTER is Owner and Director of the **Self Care Institute at Golden Apple Healing Arts**, offering holistic health care, education, and support for transformational self-care and informed health choices. She is also the Founding Director of **The Bamboo Bridge**, an international organization dedicated to the promotion of peace and health through cultural diplomacy and the harmonious integration of indigenous knowledge and new science through education and research. Dr. Libster is the national award-winning historian of *Herbal Diplomats*, a book about herbalism, nursing, and American health care reform. She has authored numerous publications including her newest book *Science of Energy Flow®- Foot Reflexology with Herbal Stress Relief* (2014), which details her 30 years as a practitioner and master teacher of the healing traditions of foot reflexology, zone therapy, and topical herbal applications. Her book *The Nurse-Herbalist: Integrative Insights for Holistic Practice* (2012) in which she weaves entertaining stories of her "partnerships" with plants with the details of a cutting-edge practice model based on nursing science and Traditional Chinese Medicine has been adopted in herbal and naturopathic schools as well as nursing education programs around the world. She is recognized internationally for her work as an Herbal Diplomat®—an expert on the complementarity of nursing practice, technology and healing traditions, in particular the use of herbal therapies.

Dr. Libster is a Board-Certified Advanced Practice Holistic Nurse and Psychiatric Mental Health Clinical Nurse Specialist in which she specializes in the care of infants age 0-5 and their caregivers. She has also practiced as a clinician-consultant in Traditional Chinese Herbal Medicine (TCM) and European and Western herbal therapies for over 25 years. Dr. Libster uses her extensive knowledge of health pattern recognition in TCM and nursing science to formulate teas and other remedies specific to her clients' needs. She cares for individuals, families, and organizations. Dr. Libster focuses her botanical practice on the application of herbal and floral teas, syrups, and topical remedies and, in addition, teaches her clients to make their own simple "medicines" for application in transformational self-care. Dr. Libster is also known for her innovations in online and tele-health care and coaching, education programs and health resource centers.

Dr. Libster is a dynamic teacher who in her 15 years in higher education has inspired new dimensions in ways of thinking about the healing arts and sciences, nursing, education, and health care reform. She offers educational opportunities, such as **Herbal Diplomat**®—a comprehensive certification program on holistic care, international health coaching, cultural diplomacy, and global health reform for the public and health clinicians. She is currently Professor of Nursing at Milwaukee School of Engineering School of Nursing where she directs the Psychiatric Mental Health Nurse Practioner Program. Dr. Libster has been a featured speaker for such organizations as the World Health Organization, the Royal College of Nursing, the International Association for Human Caring, Asian-Pacific International Conference on Complementary Nursing, and the United States Botanic Garden. She lives in Illinois, USA with her husband of 20 years and her two West Highland White Terrier pups.

Science of Energy Flow® RESOURCES

Golden Apple Healing Arts offers a number of resources to help you make the most of the Science of Energy Flow® with your clients and in your life.

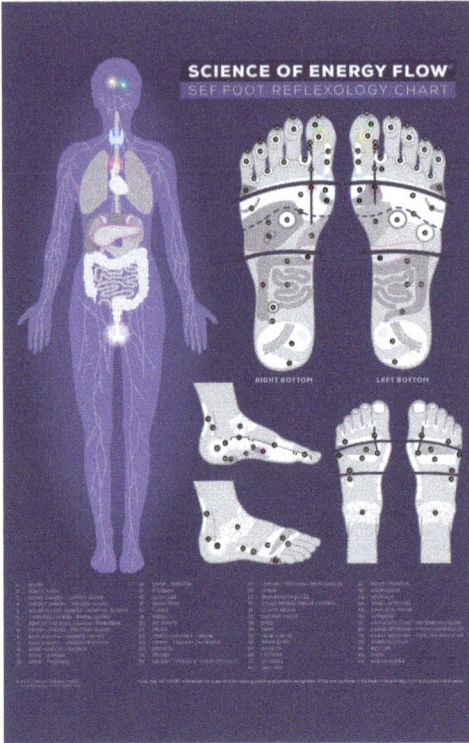

SCIENCE OF ENERGY FLOW
SEF FOOT REFLEXOLOGY CHART

Science of Energy Flow®
WALL CHART

Dr. Martha M. Libster developed this wall chart as the result of her work in anatomy and physiology, foot reflexology, Foot Zone Therapy and working with hundreds of pairs of feet of all shapes and sizes since 1984.

Features:

- Durable 18x28 inch vinyl chart suitable for display.

- Numbered key for organs and body systems.

- Seven major glands shown on body and feet in color corresponding to associated chakra

- Foot views showing top, bottom, inner, and outer feet with numbered organs for easy identification.

Science of Energy Flow®
TAU SPIRAL CHAKRA MEDITATION POSTER

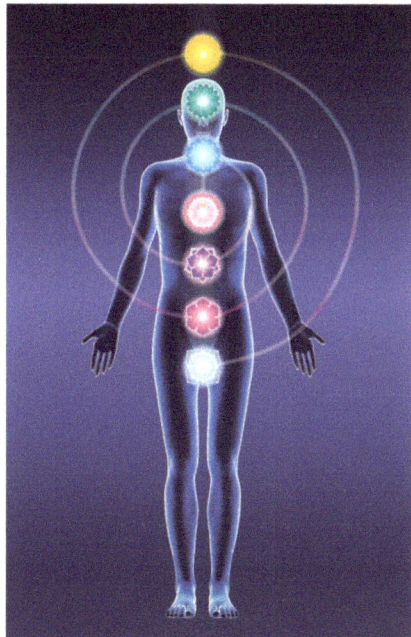

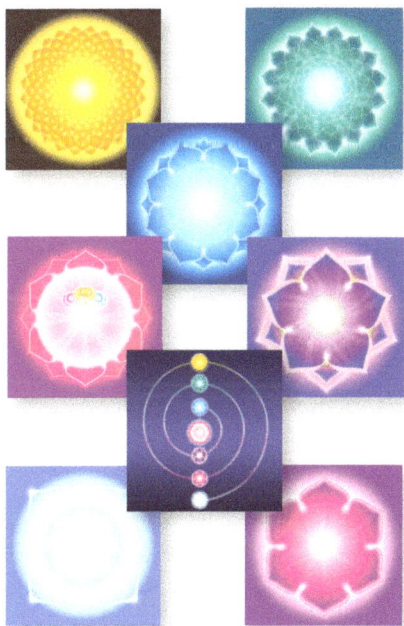

Science of Energy Flow®
TAU SPIRAL CHAKRA CARDS

The basic SEF treatment uses the seven major energy centers in the body, called Chakras. These seven colorful Chakra Cards aid in your meditation and visualization of the energy flow in the body. Set includes Tau Spiral Chakra Meditation Card.

PLEASE VISIT US AT
WWW.GOLDENAPPLEHEALINGARTS.COM
FOR DETAILS AND ORDERING.

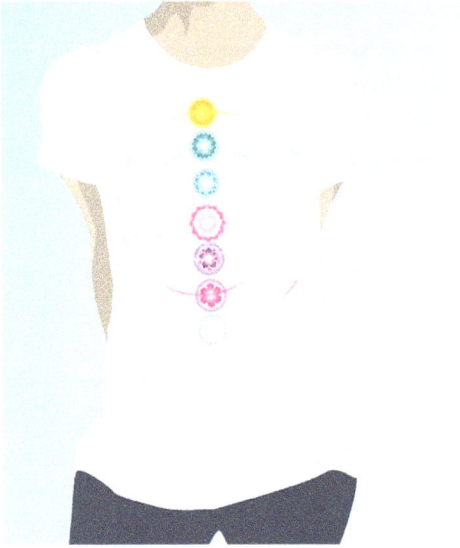

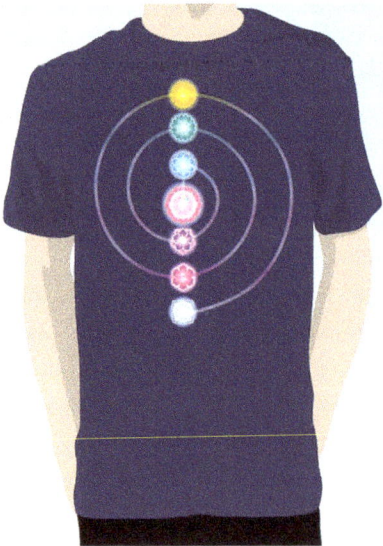

Science of Energy Flow®
TAU SPIRAL CHAKRA T-SHIRTS

These eye-catching T-shirts colorfully show the Tau Spiral connecting with the Seven chakras. The shirts were designed using the principles of Science of Energy Flow® to not just be a shirt, but a work of art and healing energy. In your choice of color, these shirts are available in your choice of Men and Women's styles and fabrics.

Product:

- Printed in color
- Size small, medium, large, Xtra-large

Science of Energy Flow®
COURSE

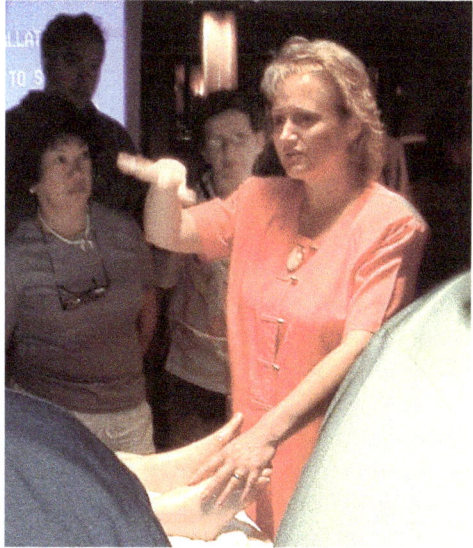

Learn more about the Science of Energy Flow® with Dr. Martha M. Libster in a face-to-face educational retreat. These retreats include the study of simple techniques for affecting correction in the energy field with the use of herbs, essential oils, and water, and the "tuning" of health patterns through the feet – Foot Reflexology. This course develops your skills in creating and maintaining healing environments of power, beauty, and protection while learning how to assist others in transmuting habits that resist well-being. Attendees will design a practice plan for the integration of techniques learned in practice (licensed attendees) and self/family care (unlicensed attendees). This hands-on course is for anyone seeking new techniques for demonstrating care to self and others.

Continuing education contact hours available. For more information and a schedule of The Science of Energy Flow® courses with Dr. Martha, please visit us at www.scienceofenergyflow.com.

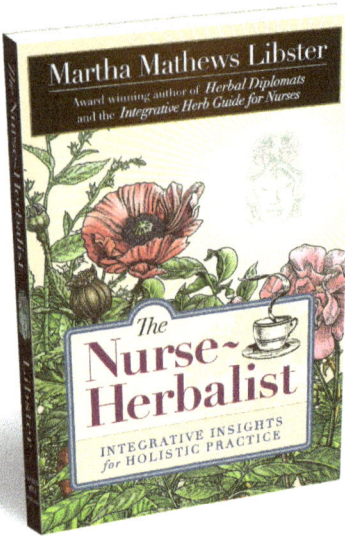

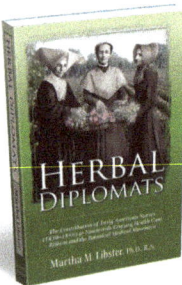

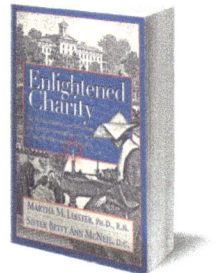

www.ingramcontent.com/pod-product-compliance
Lightning Source LLC
Chambersburg PA
CBHW052010030426
42334CB00029BA/3162